Auditory Stimulus - Response Control

Auditory Stimulus-Response Control

Edited by

Robert T. Fulton, Ph.D.

Director of Research,
Parsons Research Center,
Parsons, Kansas
and
Associate Professor,
Speech Pathology and Audiology,
University of Kansas,
Lawrence, Kansas

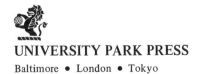

UNIVERSITY PARK PRESS

Baltimore • London • Tokyo

University Park Press
International Publishers in Science and Medicine
Chamber of Commerce Building
Baltimore, Maryland 21202

Printed in the United States of America by The Maple Press Company

Library of Congress Cataloging in Publication Data

Fulton, Robert T
  Auditory stimulus-response control.

  1. Audiometry. 2. Mentally handicapped children—
Testing. I. Title. [DNLM: 1. Audiometry—Hearing
tests—Mental retardation. WV272 F974ae]
RF294.F84   617.8'9   74-9654
ISBN 0-8391-0685-8

Contents

List of Contributors

Robert T. Fulton, Ph.D. Director of Research, Parsons Research Center (a unit of the Kansas Center for Mental Retardation and Human Development, cooperatively sponsored by the Bureau of Child Research, University of Kansas, and Parsons State Hospital and Training Center), Parsons, Kansas; and Associate Professor, Speech Pathology and Audiology, University of Kansas, Lawrence, Kansas.

Robert Hoyt, M.S. Associate Director for Communications, Bureau of Child Research, University of Kansas, Lawrence, Kansas.

James Jerger, Ph.D. Professor and Head, Division of Audiology and Speech Pathology, Baylor College of Medicine, Texas Medical Center, Houston, Texas.

Joseph E. Spradlin, Ph.D. Research Associate, Bureau of Child Research; and Professor, Human Development and Family Life, University of Kansas, Lawrence, Kansas.

Paul A. Waryas, Ph.D. Research Associate, Parsons Research Center, Kansas Center for Mental Retardation and Human Development, Parsons, Kansas.

Riley C. Worthy, M.S. Chief, Electronics Laboratory, Parsons Research Center, Kansas Center for Mental Retardation and Human Development, Parsons, Kansas.

Preface

Audiologists are typically "myth-bound." Their allegiance to ancient proverbs and unproven assumptions is legendary. Time-honored "truths" are handed down from instructor to graduate student intact and unsullied by changes in the outside world. Children suffer most from this antediluvian outlook. Students still are taught that puretones are too "abstract" for the perceptual mechanisms of young children, that "environmental" sounds are better suited to their auditory capacities. In most service facilities, the ultimate refinement in behavioral technology is to present these environmental symphonies in a "sound-field" and to judge whether the child jumped, wiggled, or grunted appropriately. Indeed, at this writing, it is possible to enter newborn infant wards of hospitals in several large cities and observe serious investigators aiming high-intensity "warbles" at sleeping babies who in all probability would have been better off left asleep.

This book is exciting to me for two reasons: first, because it demolishes so many myths and "old wive's tales" about difficult-to-test patients; second, because it shows what can be accomplished when a well-conceived, rigorously defined experimental concept is applied to a clinical problem.

Dr. Fulton and his colleagues at the Parsons Research Center carried out the bulk of this work on the mentally retarded. However, the implications of their pioneering efforts extend far beyond this single "difficult-to-test" group. Their work implies, for example, that when a child fails to respond to puretones, the fault is probably in our techniques rather than in the inability of the child to cope with "abstract" signals. Similarly, the concept that test paradigms must be confined to exceedingly simple-minded responses to loud sounds probably reflects the myopia of our clinical approach rather than the inability of the child to respond meaningfully to more complex stimuli.

The enormity of what these dedicated investigators have accomplished hardly can be overstated. As the reader progresses through this volume, he will find nonverbal subjects (with IQ's as low as 12) being trained to produce valid and reliable puretone responses, to perform the short-increment sensitivity index and tone decay test, and to execute incredibly sophisticated psychophysical judgments of minimal detectable increments in frequency, intensity, and time. The contrast between this level of sophistication and what passes for pediatric evaluation in many audiology centers today is truly staggering.

Over and above its immediate clinical implications, however, this book provides a challenging model for the welding of "clinical" and "research" audiologists. We hear the frequent, and usually justified, criticism that clinicians continue traditions passed on from one generation to the next in total oblivion of significant advances in research, while dilettante researchers labor over minutia in splendid isolation from the real world.

What Fulton and his colleagues have done is to show how rather basic research findings in two areas—operant conditioning and the theory of signal detectability—can be applied to a very real clinical problem, obtaining audiograms on subjects with limited verbal skills. In so doing, they have made an immeasurable contribution to our field.

It is instructive, therefore, to examine their strategy. The most striking observation I make is that one searches in vain for the traditional dichotomy between researcher and clinician. We do not find researchers developing the techniques in the laboratory, then delivering them to the clinician for "field trial." We find, instead, that it is impossible to tell who is the researcher and who is the clinician. Indeed, they are one and the same person. Fulton and his team are both researcher and clinician. In every chapter, we find them developing a technique, trying it out on real patients, modifying it as a result of actual clinical trial, and then starting over. The researcher is the clinician. The clinician is the researcher. There is a valuable lesson here. I hope it is not lost.

James Jerger, Ph.D.
Houston, Texas

Acknowledgments

This work was supported by grants from the National Institute of Child Health and Human Development (HD-00870, HD-02528, and HD-05088) and the National Institute of Mental Health (MH-14877).

A significant charitable contribution to our psychoacoustic calibration and stimulus analyses instrumentation array was made by Tektronix Incorporated, Beaverton, Oregon.

These investigations could not have been completed without the support of many persons not credited with authorship: families, colleagues, research assistants, research support personnel, and subjects. The authors are grateful to all who helped through their various channels.

The editor extends his thanks to John F. Brandt, Lyle L. Lloyd, and Riley C. Worthy, who spent many hours reading and advising, and to Richard L. Schiefelbusch, Director of the Bureau of Child Research, University of Kansas, and Howard V. Bair, Superintendent, Parsons State Hospital and Training Center, for their administrative support.

Significant technical contributions were made by: Cheryl Burzinski, Ross Copeland, Pamela Gorzycki, Peggy Hartman, Dennie Hurt, Michael J. Reid, J. D. Sexton, Ruth Staten, and by the staff of the Parsons State Hospital and Training Center Audio-Visual Department and the Media Support System of the University of Kansas (at Parsons), Bureau of Child Research.

Special Acknowledgments

The editor is particularly indebted to six persons who have had tremendous influence on his career and who have made this line of investigation and this writing possible, exciting, and pleasurable:

Joseph Spradlin, mentor, colleague, consultant, and friend. He has been instrumental in the thrust of the editor's research career.

Robert Hoyt, teacher, colleague, and friend. He has provided the impetus for communicating research and research ideas. He also served as technical editor for this work.

Paul Waryas, a colleague who added an element of cooperative research that few investigators have the opportunity to experience.

James Jerger, mentor and consultant. He made significant contributions to the direction of this writing and provided a necessary final burst of enthusiasm for its completion.

Riley Worthy, whose skill in instrumentation made these experiments possible.

Wilma Hull, who served as the editor's research assistant for five years. She collected the major portion of the data in this work and served in every other possible capacity (statistical clerk, graphics technician, secretary, etc.), and provided a continuous stabilizing effect through what often were hectic times.

RTF

Robert T. Fulton and
Joseph E. Spradlin # Introduction

LIMITATIONS IN CURRENT APPROACHES

Information concerning the auditory system of a child may have implications for both medical and educational treatment. Yet, in the case of children with language handicaps, the handicap may interfere with attempts to evaluate the auditory system. Severely retarded, autistic, aphasic, deaf, and very young normal children may fail to follow test directions required to produce reliable and valid information concerning the condition of their auditory systems. Since such children may not respond well to typical methods of instruction, they often receive incomplete or inadequate evaluations. For example, an evaluation may state that "the child initially responded to the examiner's voice but no audiometric tests could be made," or, "no response to loud sounds occurred; however, it could not be determined whether this was due to a severe hearing loss or to the child's autistic condition." If an examiner cannot determine whether there is a hearing loss, then it usually is not possible to administer more refined and diagnostically definitive tests.

Recent work on cortical-evoked responses (Goldstein, 1973; Price, 1969; Skinner, 1972) and impedance procedures (Fulton and Lamb, 1972; Lamb and Norris, 1969; Lilly, 1972, 1973) holds promise for evaluation of such children, but even these procedures are more useful with cooperative subjects than with those described above. Current cortical-evoked response and impedance procedures yield valuable information concerning the auditory system, but they do not present a total picture of processing of auditory stimuli by children.

THE IMPORTANCE OF RELIABLE TESTING

We often rationalize our failure to obtain reliable and valid information by saying that, compared with his other problems, it is unimportant whether or not a severely developmentally deficient child hears. Medically and educationally, it does make a difference. Retarded children are known to have a higher incidence of otologic pathology than do normal subjects (Fulton and Griffin, 1967; Fulton and Lloyd, 1968; Pantalakos, 1963). Therefore, if for no other reason, it is important to the child's health if a pathologic condition exists. If his auditory system is intact, it may be possible to train the child to respond appropriately to speech stimuli. If the system is not intact, he may still profit from medical treatment, amplification, or programs for teaching him other forms of language.

The problems of a severely retarded, autistic, deaf, or aphasic child may be compounded by a parent, teacher, or language therapist who is trying to teach the child without knowing whether or not he has functional hearing.

There are those who ask, "why bother to evaluate the auditory system of difficult-to-test persons when one can accomplish so much more with others?" There is some validity in such a question. Developing assessment and training procedures for the difficult-to-test is demanding and time-consuming. Evaluations, even under ideal conditions, take longer than with other persons. Also, with most difficult-to-test persons, changes in behavior take hours of training even after surgical intervention or fitting with an amplification device. However, the issue of taking time to develop procedures for evaluating and training the difficult-to-test is a value judgment, and as in all value judgments, arguments and counter-arguments are plentiful and inconclusive.

REASONS FOR GENERALIZING THE PROCEDURES

The retarded and the autistic have enough problems without the additional liability of an undetected auditory handicap.

Not all difficult-to-test persons are pathologically deficient or demonstrate noncontrollable behaviors. Young children (less than 3 years old) are among the most difficult to evaluate. Since adequate hearing is critical to language development, early information on hearing is especially important if a child shows a delay in speech or language development. Early detection of a hearing loss can lead to the use of amplification, to surgery, or to the removal of those obstructions from the environment which preclude the child from normal development.

Equally important is the need to understand the responses of children to auditory stimuli and to develop programs for training communication skills. The study of responses to basic acoustic stimuli can lead to auditory discrimination programs and subsequently to improved communication skills.

Shortcomings in obtaining precise auditory information on severely handicapped children are unjustified when we consider that we have developed procedures for obtaining precise auditory information on lower animals (Clack and Herman, 1963; Dalland, 1965; Heffner, Ravizza, and Masterton, 1969a,b; Heffner, Heffner, and Masterton, 1971; Ravizza, Heffner, and Masterton, 1969a,b; Wollack, 1963). Recent research clearly indicates that procedures similar to those used in animal research are applicable to the evaluation of handicapped children (Bricker and Bricker, 1969; Fulton and Spradlin, 1971; LaCrosse and Bidlake, 1964; Lloyd, Spradlin, and Reid, 1968; Meyerson and Michael, 1960; Spradlin et al., 1968; Spradlin, Locke, and Fulton, 1969).

PURPOSE OF THIS WORK

There are three main goals for this publication:
1. To describe the basic mechanics and procedures for assessing the auditory system of severely handicapped and difficult-to-test children.
2. To demonstrate the application of these procedures in the clinical (audiometric) and basic (psychoacoustic) auditory assessment of these children.
3. To provide clinical and basic assessment data which can be used to develop better assessment procedures and to develop programs for training communication skills.

The material presented here is characterized by the application of behavioral principles to obtain precise control over the responses of children and by the use of audiologic and acoustic information to determine precisely what stimulus change was controlling the child's response. Chapter 1 presents the principles and strategies involved in obtaining stimulus-response control, while Chapter 2 evaluates these training procedures. Chapters 3–5 present the "Applications to Audiometric Technology" and discuss the application and resultant clinical data of stimulus-response control procedures to puretone thresholds (Chapter 3), the short-increment sensitivity index (Chapter 4), and the threshold tone decay test (Chapter 5). Chapters 6–8, "Applications to Psychoacoustic Research," discuss investigations of three basic psychoacoustic parameters (time, frequency, and intensity) with difficult-to-test and normal subjects.

The psychoacoustic section is particularly significant in that it presents the first known psychoacoustic research with retarded children. If information on the audiologic assessment of retarded children is limited, information on auditory detection and processing is even more so. Much of the information presented is relevant to auditory perception.

The final section summarizes and attempts to identify areas in which further investigation is needed. The "Appendices" contain technical information (detailed plans and schematics for all instrumentation used in this research) which is too cumbersome to handle in the text.

THE BASIS OF THIS WORK

Although the procedures described here are applicable to other organisms and other populations, we restrict our discussion to children. A few basic principles figure very prominently in this work.

1. **Children are active and exhibit a variety of behaviors.** We do not know the source of the behaviors that all children exhibit, but they do occur. This is true even for severely handicapped children. These behaviors are *operant responses*.

2. **When certain events immediately follow a specific type of behavior, the probability that this behavior will reoccur increases.** These events are *reinforcers*. If an event which is presented contingent on responses increases their rate or probability, it is a *positive reinforcer*. Positive reinforcers are usually pleasant things, such as smiles, hugs, or sweets. However, they need not be. If, when a child picks his nose, a parent scolds the child for this behavior and the rate of nose-picking increases, the "parent scolds" are positive reinforcers for that child.

3. **If a response is reinforced in the presence of a specific environmental feature (discriminative stimulus), the response probability will increase when that environmental feature is present.** Conversely, if the response never is reinforced when that feature is absent, the probability that a response will occur when the feature is absent will decrease. For example, if a child is reinforced for making a response only when a stimulus is present, he will respond more when the stimulus is present than when it is absent.

4. **Reinforcing events are dependent on the state of the child.** For example, chocolate candy is a much more effective reinforcer if the child has not eaten immediately before the candy is used as a reinforcing agent. This principle is especially important to remember if long sessions are used. Otherwise, the child may become satiated during the session.

While the four principles listed above are remarkably simple, their application in the development of an effective audiometric procedure for evaluating the auditory system of handicapped children is not so simple. It is difficult to select a response which most children can make yet which clearly identifies a discrete response from other varying behaviors. The novice experimenter may spend considerable time arriving at a discrete response which is easy for the child to make.

SELECTING AND DELIVERING REINFORCEMENT

It is sometimes difficult to find an effective edible reinforcer for a specific child. This is especially true if the clinician has no control over the child's diet. Many training plans have failed because the clinician could not find an effective reinforcer or did not make sure that the reinforcer was effective throughout the program.

Immediate delivery of reinforcement is equally difficult. Delivering reinforcement 10, 5, or even 2 seconds after the response may require a prolonged training procedure. It is often difficult to deliver an edible, a hug, or drink of juice immediately. For this reason, a light and/or a chime may be delivered immediately after the child makes a correct response. Such stimuli bridge the gap between the response and the reinforcement.

The physical state of the child is also difficult to control if the examiner has no influence over food and liquid intake. Moreover, drugs administered to control convulsions or behavior disorders may interfere with performance. In our experiments, we did not control the child's food, liquid, or drug intake. However, we did attempt to develop procedures for evaluating the daily reliability and validity of our procedures, and thus we excluded data recorded on days when children were satiated, drugged so heavily that they could not be controlled, or ill.

The practice of reinforcing a response in the presence of a stimulus and not reinforcing the response when the stimulus is not present seems simple. If the subject responds at a high rate, even when the stimulus is absent, and then is reinforced for his first response when the stimulus is presented, discrimination has not been developed. Under these conditions, a chain of behaviors may be established which are incompatible with differential responding to the stimulus. Also, if the subject responds just as the stimulus is presented and before he has an opportunity to perceive it, he has been reinforced functionally for an incorrect response.

All of these problems influence the hearing evaluation of any severely handicapped child. There are even greater problems with children who have severe hearing losses. How can the clinician be certain that the failure to obtain stimulus control is due to a hearing loss rather than to procedural inadequacies? And, since the control by the auditory stimulus is not an all-or-nothing process, what assurance is there that the subject is responding discriminatively rather than randomly?

The following chapters, notably Chapter 1, "Basic Stimulus-Response Control Training Procedures," present an approach for solving these problems.

DEVELOPING RESEARCH PROCEDURES

Most research reports imply a very orderly plan with explicit criteria for accepting results as valid and for introducing changes in procedures. During the developmental stages of our work, such orderliness was rarely apparent. We used small numbers of children, usually never more than four and sometimes only one, to determine whether a child could be conditioned to the point at which we could obtain stimulus-response control. We usually changed procedures several times before we were able to obtain adequate stimulus-response control. Often, midpoint in a procedure, we saw things we did not like about the response mechanism and changed it immediately. There were no t tests to determine whether the response mechanism really was related to the child's failure to make a clean discrete response. We simply assumed that it might be improved and we introduced the change. After each child or set of children had been examined, we designed a procedure and tried to follow it through with a new subject. At times during the first session with the first child, a new problem arose. The program was changed again and again. After we developed an instrumented program, we often overrode the program with manual controls, thinking, usually correctly, that we could do better than the instrumentation. Each time we made such a manual adjustment, we attempted to build that adjustment into the program. That is, each time we thought we had learned something, we modified the instrumentation, which often exercised better control after the program change. Our initial recording of responses was clinical, that is, the clinician decided whether the child responded to the signal or by chance. Later, however, we worked out an instrumented recording procedure which made those judgments easier. By the time 40 or 50 children had been tested, we had developed an almost totally automated program which was effective for more than 85 percent of the children tested.

BROADENING THE RESEARCH AREA

As we gained experience, we expanded the range of hearing phenomena under investigation. Our first goal was to obtain air-conduction tests. Previous work in this area had been conducted by Lloyd et al. (1968). We expanded on that initial work, examining bone-conduction tests, masking, and other tests such as the short-increment sensitivity index (SISI) and the threshold tone decay test. That led us to reconceptualize our problems and change our procedures.

Since some latter tests involved a continuous acoustic signal, we realized that we must conceptualize the task not as a simple "stimulus detection" process but as a "stimulus change detection" process. Thus, we changed our initial training task to include a signal superimposed on a band of noise or pedestal tone rather than the presentation of a signal on a background of silence (ambient noise). Subjects trained with this procedure rapidly generalized from tasks involving puretone air-conduction threshold tests to bone-conduction tests, masked thresholds, SISI tests, tone decay tests, and finally to psychoacoustic tests of frequency and intensity change or duration detection.

The current basic procedure requires a single detection response to a change in the auditory input. This procedure appears ideal as a first step in the evaluation of handicapped children because results derived by it are relatively unaffected by cortical lesions (Elliott and Trahiotis, 1972).

THE REPORTING STYLE

Several sections depart from traditional research reporting for a style of presentation in which the procedures illustrate the application of the principles and the results support the propositions under investigation. In this way, we hope to inform readers who are new to these principles and procedures, to suggest procedures for the clinically oriented reader, and at the same time to provide data for the research-oriented reader.

We have not included a comprehensive review of the audiologic literature with the retarded or difficult-to-test. Several reviews already cover the area (Fulton and Lloyd, 1969; Webb and Kinde, 1967; Lloyd, 1970; Lloyd and Moore, 1972; Rittmanic, 1971). Frisina (1973) and Hodgson (1972) discuss the problems of evaluating infants and young children. Psychoacoustic research with the retarded is conspicuously absent in the literature. We have attempted to limit the relevant psychoacoustic literature from research with normal subjects to that specifically related to the discussion at hand and have refrained from in-depth discussions of acoustic theory.

We have tried to adhere to classical psychophysical methods, standard audiometric procedural principles, and sound experimental design. Modifications were limited to procedural necessity where principles permitted.

Throughout this book, we have referred to the adaptive behavior and/or measured intelligence levels of subjects under investigation. The levels and their respective references were effective at the time that the studies were being conducted. However, the reader should be aware of a more recent discussion of the area (Grossman, 1973) and is referred to it.

SUMMARY

There are many children and adults who, because of various behavioral problems, resist or defy traditional auditory assessment and training procedures and as a result go unattended. Their educational and medical needs are as critical as those of persons who do not exhibit aberrant behaviors.

The principles underlying behavior control, combined with the precision of sound clinical and research practices, provide a mechanism for evaluating and training these difficult-to-test persons. The precision of managing human behavior is equally as important for the attainment of reliable information as the precision that usually is accorded the control of auditory stimuli.

The assertion that the retarded, young children, or a variety of other difficult-to-test populations are incapable of responding to "abstract signals such as puretones" is refuted by the data throughout this document. That assertion arises from a failure to attain stimulus-response control through training and not because of the acoustic properties of the stimulus or the related perceptual skills of etiological or behavioral populations.

This book attempts to provide the basis for developing and applying the basic principles of both behavioral control and precise acoustic stimulus specification to the study of audition. In no way should it be inferred that the procedures presented here are the ultimate in such management. However, in view of the current status of auditory assessment and training procedures with difficult-to-test persons, the acceptance of these procedures by professionals working with these populations will make this work significant. If the reader extends these procedures and applications beyond the examples presented, thus outdating the examples, this work will have been successful.

LITERATURE CITED

Bricker, D., and W. A. Bricker. 1969. A programmed approach to operant audiometry for low functioning children. J. Speech Hear. Dis. 34: 312–320.

Clack, T. D., and P. N. Herman. 1963. A single-lever psychophysical adjustment procedure for measuring auditory thresholds in the monkey. J. Audit. Res. 3: 175–183.

Dalland, J. I. 1965. Auditory thresholds in the bat: A behavioral technique. J. Audit. Res. 5: 95–108.

Elliott, D. N., and C. Trahiotis. 1972. Cortical lesions and auditory discrimination. Psychol. Bull. 3: 198–222.

Frisina, R. 1973. Measurement of hearing in children. In: J. Jerger (ed.), Modern Developments in Audiology, pp. 155–174. 2nd Ed. Academic Press, New York.

Fulton, R. T., and C. S. Griffin. 1967. Audiological-otological considerations with the mentally retarded. Ment. Retard. 5: 26–31.

Fulton, R. T., and L. E. Lamb. 1972. Acoustic impedance and tympanometry with the retarded: A normative study. Audiology 11: 199–208.

Fulton, R. T., and L. L. Lloyd. 1968. Hearing impairment in a population of children with Down's syndrome. Amer. J. Ment. Defic. 73:298–302.

Fulton, R. T., and L. L. Lloyd (eds.). 1969. Audiometry for the Retarded: With Implications for the Difficult-to-Test. Williams & Wilkins, Baltimore.

Fulton, R. T., and J. E. Spradlin. 1971. Operant audiometry with severely retarded children. Audiology 10: 203–211.

Goldstein, R. 1973. Electroencephalic audiometry. In: J. Jerger (ed.), Modern Developments in Audiology, pp. 407–435. 2nd Ed. Academic Press, New York.

Grossman, H. J. (ed.). 1973. Manual on Terminology and Classification in Mental Retardation. Revised ed. American Association on Mental Deficiency, Washington, D. C.

Heffner, H. E., R. J. Ravizza, and B. Masterton. 1969a. Hearing in primitive mammals. III. Tree shrew. J. Audit. Res. 9: 12–18.

Heffner, H. E., R. J. Ravizza, and B. Masterton. 1969b. Hearing in primitive mammals. IV. Bushbaby. J. Audit. Res. 9: 19–23.

Heffner, R., H. Heffner, and B. Masterton. 1971. Behavioral measurements of absolute and frequency difference thresholds in guinea pig. J. Acoust. Soc. Amer. 49: 1888–1895.

Hodgson, W. R. 1972. Testing infants and young children. In: J. Katz (ed.), Handbook of Clinical Audiology, pp. 498–519. Williams & Wilkins, Baltimore.

LaCrosse, E. L., and H. Bidlake. 1964. A method to test the hearing of mentally retarded children. Volta Rev. 66: 27–30.

Lamb, L. E., and T. W. Norris. 1969. Acoustic impedance measurement. In: R. T. Fulton and L. L. Lloyd (eds.), Audiometry for the Retarded: With Implications for the Difficult-to-Test, pp. 196–209. Williams & Wilkins, Baltimore.

Lilly, D. J. 1972. Acoustic impedance at the tympanic membrane. In: J. Katz (ed.), Handbook of Clinical Audiology, pp. 434–469. Williams & Wilkins, Baltimore.

Lilly, D. J. 1973. Measurement of acoustic impedance at the tympanic membrane. In: J. Jerger (ed.), Modern Developments in Audiology, pp. 345–406. 2nd Ed. Academic Press, New York.

Lloyd, L. L. 1970. Audiologic aspects of mental retardation. In: N. R. Ellis (ed.), International Review of Mental Retardation. Vol. 4, pp. 311–363. Academic Press, New York.

Lloyd, L. L., and E. J. Moore. 1972. Audiology. In: J. Wortis (ed.), Mental Retardation: An Annual Review. Vol 4, pp. 141–163. Grune & Stratton, New York.

Lloyd, L. L., J. E. Spradlin, and M. J. Reid. 1968. An operant audiometric procedure for difficult-to-test patients. J. Speech Hear. Dis. 33: 236–245.

Meyerson, L., and J. L. Michael. 1960. The measurement of sensory thresholds in exceptional children: An experimental approach to some problems of differential diagnosis and education with special reference to hearing.

Cooperative Research Project No. 418. U. S. Office of Education, Dept. of Health, Education, and Welfare, University of Houston, Houston, Texas.

Pantalakos, C. G. 1963. Audiometric and otolaryngologic survey of retarded students. N. C. Med. J. 24: 238–242.

Price, L. L. 1969. Cortical-evoked response audiometry. *In:* R. T. Fulton and L. L. Lloyd (eds.), Audiometry for the Retarded: With Implications for the Difficult-to-Test, pp. 210–237. Williams & Wilkins, Baltimore.

Ravizza, R. J., H. E. Heffner, and B. Masterton. 1969a. Hearing in primitive mammals. I. Opossum. J. Audit. Res. 9: 1–7.

Ravizza, R. J:, H. E. Heffner, and B. Masterton. 1969b. Hearing in primitive mammals. II. Hedgehog. J. Audit. Res. 9: 8–11.

Rittmanic, P. 1971. The mentally retarded and mentally ill. *In:* D. Rose (ed.), Audiological Assessment, pp. 369–404. Prentice-Hall, Englewood Cliffs, N. J.

Skinner, P. H. 1972. Electroencephalic response audiometry. *In:* J. Katz (ed.), Handbook of Clinical Audiology, pp. 407–433. Williams & Wilkins, Baltimore.

Spradlin, J. E., L. L. Lloyd, G. L. Hom, and M. J. Reid. 1968. Establishing tone control and evaluating the hearing of severely retarded children. *In:* G. A. Jervis (ed.), Expanding Concepts in Mental Retardation, pp. 170–180. Charles C Thomas, Springfield, Ill.

Spradlin, J. E., B. J. Locke, and R. T. Fulton. 1969. Conditioning and audiological assessment. *In:* R. T. Fulton and L. L. Lloyd (eds.), Audiometry for the Retarded: With implications for the Difficult-to-Test, pp. 125–163. Williams & Wilkins, Baltimore.

Webb, C. E., and S. Kinde. 1967. Speech, language and hearing of the mentally retarded. *In:* A. A. Baumeister (ed.), Mental Retardation, pp. 86–119. Aldine Publishing Co., Chicago.

Wollack, C. H. 1963. The auditory acuity of the sheep (*Ovis aries*). J. Audit. Res. 3: 121–132.

Establishing Stimulus-Response Control

Information is only as valid and reliable as the means by which it was obtained. So it is also with the auditory assessment of difficult-to-test persons. If a clinician or experimenter is unable to examine his assessment data with confidence, the tenet of his work has been violated. He must ensure, to the best of his ability, that the data were obtained under maximally controlled conditions. This control is equally as important in obtaining subject responses as it is in controlling the parameters of the stimulus.

This section is designed to assist in the establishment of control of the subject's response to the stimulus.

1 Basic Stimulus - Response Control Training Procedures

Robert T. Fulton and Joseph E. Spradlin

DEFINITION OF TRAINING PROCEDURES

The procedures used in this work are based on an operant or instrumental conditioning model. This model is commonly diagrammed as: *Stimulus → Response → Reinforcement.* In the usual stimulus → response (S → R) model, the subject is presented with an auditory stimulus, and if he makes some response (such as holding up his hand), we say he hears the signal. When the subject is a normal adult or an older child, obtaining such a response presents no problem. The audiologist simply instructs the subject to hold up his hand each time he hears the signal. It is assumed that, under such instructions, the stimulus-response relationship is so firmly established that if the subject does not make the prescribed response, he did not hear the signal. Since normal persons respond so consistently to directions before coming to the audiometric situation, we often pay little attention to the final component of the model—namely, reinforcement. When dealing with young children or difficult-to-test patients, such an oversight often leads to invalid audiometric information. Since the difficult-to-test child does not follow instructions reliably, we must devise special procedures for bringing his responses under stimulus-response control (see Appendix A). This chapter provides a description of the procedures for bringing a child's responses under the control of auditory stimuli. The procedures include identifying a practical reinforcer, developing a discrete response, and bringing that response under the control of an auditory stimulus.

REINFORCEMENT

The use of reinforcement in audiologic procedures is not new. However, most previous applications have not been systematic. One shortcoming of past uses has been the failure to select or establish a functional reinforcer. Events which serve as reinforcers are highly individualized. An event or item is not a reinforcer until it has been so defined by the subject. Reinforcers are not determined by the examiner. Candy is a reinforcer for some children and not for others. The same can be said of social contact, beverages, and nearly all other agents which at one time or another have been used as reinforcers. Effectiveness is especially limited if the child has not been deprived of the reinforcer before initiation of the testing session. Many instrumental conditioning techniques of the past would have been much more effective and received greater acceptance if the basic principles of reinforcement had been understood and greater effort had been expended in determining an effective reinforcer for each child tested.

Lloyd (1966) was one of the first to emphasize the extent and application of reinforcement principles to behavioral audiometry. Considerable success has been achieved with the use of edibles as reinforcers, particularly with young and severely retarded children. Candy is used often in conditioning studies with children. There are three principle reasons for the wide use of candy. First, it is reinforcing to most children. Second, it is easily dispensed. Third, practitioners have been notoriously uncreative in developing other types of reinforcers. However, not all children like candy, or, for that matter, other edibles. One subject rejected test conditions and at times became violent unless the reinforcing agent was candy mints or classical music (music was used in nonauditory experiments). Over a period of 5 years we have used crackers, a variety of candies, pretzels, cheese puffs, peanuts, roasted soy beans, raisins, cereal, pieces of carrots, puddings, liquids, miniature marshmallows, Metrecal (Mead Johnson & Co., Evansville, Ind.), popcorn, and ice cream.

We have used sugarless items for diabetic subjects and nonchewable items for persons with oral and/or laryngeal pathologies. At times, it has been necessary to combine edibles with social reinforcement such as patting or verbally praising the subject.

One effective means of selecting reinforcers is to use a "cafetèria" (subject selection) system. The experimenter gives the subject a variety of items one at a time and observes which items are acceptable. The experimenter then shows the subject the preferred item in the palm of his hand and closes his fist. If the subject attempts to open the closed fist, an effective reinforcer probably has been found. Another way is to display the items in a box, i.e., clear plastic "nut and bolt" case, and to ask the subject to indicate his choice by pointing to it. This latter technique is rarely useful on initial contacts, since most persons who can respond appropriately to such verbal directions also can be evaluated with more conventional audiometric techniques.

Edible material should be delivered sparingly to maintain control yet minimize satiation. Some children may respond reliably during a period in which they receive over 100 pieces of candy or food. Others may stop responding after only a few.

A reinforcer may lose its potency over a period of time; therefore, it is important to probe continuously its effectiveness and strength, on an individual level, as a reinforcing agent.

RESPONSE-REINFORCEMENT APPARATUS

The response-reinforcement delivery apparatus shown in Figures 1 and 2 is the most common reinforcement system used in our laboratories (see Appen-

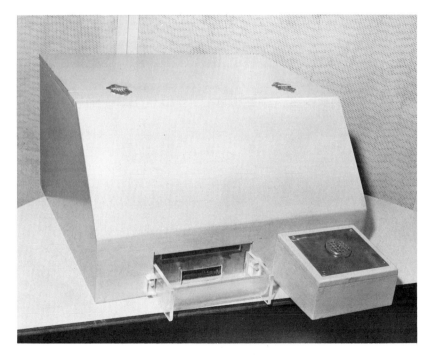

Figure 1. Response and reinforcement delivery apparatus.

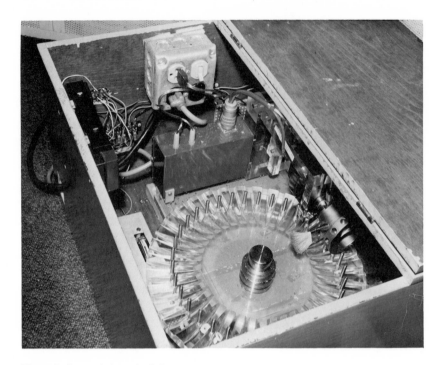

Figure 2. Internal view of reinforcement apparatus.

dix B, Plates 1 and 2 for detailed construction plans). It contains a Davis Model 310 universal feeder (Davis Scientific Instruments, N. Hollywood, Calif.) (see Figure 2). Upon an appropriate response, an edible drops into the tray, the Plexiglas area around the tray is lighted from inside the reinforcement box, and a door chime is sounded. The light and chimes serve as conditioned reinforcers, or bridging stimuli, for immediate feedback to the subject.

The tray is constructed with a round bottom to facilitate cleaning between sessions. Food may not melt or dissolve in the hand of the experimenter, but the subject's placing of food and fingers simultaneously in the mouth almost always results in a messy tray and response button by the end of the session. Cleaning and disinfecting the tray and response button after use by each subject should be standard procedure.

With automated reinforcement, it is advisable to use a dispenser such as the Davis universal feeder because of its adaptability in delivering a variety of solid agents. M & M dispensers are limited to M & M's or items of similar shape. Liquid dispensers (Davis Model LR-132) are limited to liquids, and the delivery system creates additional instrumentation problems. Although not common, liquid and food reinforcement dispensers have been used together in stereotyped behavior research (Hollis, 1973). This combination can be modified for auditory research.

Continuous reinforcement (CRF), reinforcement for each correct response, is used unless an extensive number of trials per session or a long series of sessions threatens to satiate the patient. In such cases, the ratio of reinforcement is increased gradually to avoid extinction. When ratios, either fixed or variable, are increased, the conditioned reinforcers, i.e., light and chime, continue to be activated for each correct response. The higher ratios of reinforcement serve as a limit on food consumption.

SELECTING AND DEVELOPING A RESPONSE APPARATUS

There is a tendency to react to subject responses rather casually in behavioral audiology. Localization or head-turning responses have been used in such procedures as the "Conditioned Orientation Reflex" procedure (Fulton, 1962; Liden and Kankkunen, 1969; Suzuki and Ogiba, 1960, 1961). Such responses are subject to considerable variability and examiner subjectivity and are difficult to record automatically. For convenience, and to ensure a discrete response, we have selected a button press which permits discrete responding and automatic recording.

Obtaining discrete responses across a broad range of populations offers a challenge to the examiner who has experienced initial success with his choice of manipulandum. Several procedures have used a button[1] mounted on the end of a flexible cord. This arrangement is convenient for subjects because the response button is not mounted in a fixed position. However, many children use the switch cord to "tie up" imaginary robbers or animals, or the switch to pound the furniture or themselves. The switch makes an excellent, but probably tasteless, lollipop. Fixed-position switches help to keep the subject within the immediate vicinity of the reinforcement delivery apparatus. Otherwise, the subject misses opportunities for reinforcement. Even the position of the switch in relation to other movements or activity, such as reinforcer retrieval, is important. In the early work, the investigators used a two-button arrangement (Spradlin and Lloyd, 1965) or positioned a single switch (Spradlin et al., 1968) in a central location with easy access to the reinforcement delivery tray. The switch was positioned so that the subject had no immediate resting place (table) for his hand between responses. Experience has demonstrated that the current location (see Figure 1) is the

---

[1] The terms "button," "key," and "switch" are used interchangeably in reference to the response device.

most advantageous position when using the type of reinforcing apparatus shown. In this position, the hand can rest on the table, yet is within a few inches of the button for a response. The response button is also immediately adjacent to the reinforcement delivery tray. The button is placed on the right side of the apparatus because most children are right-handed, yet it does not restrict left-handed responders. Some subjects use only one hand to press the button and retrieve the reinforcer. Others set up hand-motor patterns in which the right hand makes the response while the left hand retrieves the reinforcer. This may be the most expedient for the subject, but he may keep his right hand on the button while he is delivering the reinforcer to his mouth with his left hand. Because the equipment is programmed so that no signal is presented when the subject's hand is on the button or in the immediate area, this latter motor pattern has the advantage of providing a stimulus presentation schedule compatible with the subject's schedule of consuming the reinforcer. We continually look for and experiment with improved response and reinforcement topographies.

Selecting a Response Key

We have found the BRS Foringer Key assembly (SMR-001, nonfrosted, or SMR-002, frosted) (BRS-Foringer, Beltsville, Md.) to be a good general-purpose response button. It is sturdy and permits adjustable depression tension. Many children are not respectful of manipulanda, and sturdy construction is absolutely essential. In our attempt to evaluate new or different switches, we have found a quick and simple test. The switch is mounted on a stable base and the experimenter hits it as hard as he can with his fist. This is rather nondata-oriented, but effective. The BRS Foringer key has stood the test well. Others have gone quickly to the junk pile.

Even the BRS Foringer key requires modification. The base of the key is mounted on either a board or a heavy piece of Plexiglas, and the response pedestal shaft is raised (Plexiglas) to make it easily accessible for a quick discrete response (see Appendix B, Plate 3). Even the best response buttons occasionally need readjustment. This is particularly irritating to the examiner during a training or test session. Therefore, it is advisable to have a spare readily available. We always have two switches available for immediate interchange. Rapid interchange is accomplished by attaching automobile convertible-top snaps to the base of the response plate and installing electrical plugs (see Appendix B, Plate 4). The exchange can be completed within a matter of seconds.

The Response Area

The face of the response area, including the button, is covered with stainless steel and wired to a capacitance switch. That portion of the plate which covers the actual response button is perforated to permit light to be transmitted through the button. The perforations in the steel plate are filled with liquid plastic and polished to a smooth surface to prevent the perforations from becoming filled with dirt and food particles (see Appendix B, Plate 3). We use the term "touch plate" to identify the overall modification of the response area. Any time contact is made with the plate or button surface, a capacitance switch is activated. The capacitance switch is programmed to delay the auditory presentation program for the duration of the contact plus a predetermined penalty period ("time out"). The result is that as long as the subject nondiscriminately plays with or around the response area, the program penalizes the subject by not providing opportunities (auditory signals) for reinforcement. This modification, in conjunction with reinforcement of discriminative responses, has been effective in the training of a discrete response (a schematic diagram of a capacitance switch can be found in Appendix B, Plate 5). Subsequent to developing this switch, we have found that the U300M remote switch (Magic Dot, Minneapolis, Minn.) can be used or modified to serve the same function.

Although the button press switch has been used successfully with a 12-month-old child, some subjects respond so lightly that they do not activate the button relay. For these subjects, we have built a flat response plate, or wire screen, which is connected to the capacitance switch and which, in turn, triggers the reinforcement apparatus. This switch is particularly appropriate for infants with limited button-depressing skills; many infants are unable to generate sufficient finger or hand pressure to activate a button-press response. Nowles (1971) used a similar type of switch with 2-year-olds. However, when the response plate and capacitance switch are programmed to effect a response, the capability for controlling random nondiscriminative contact with the response area is lost.

Although we never have attempted to develop a response switch which retains the contact time-out consequences yet which permits a touch response to effect a reinforced discrimination, it appears to be possible to do so. During intertrial periods, the switch could serve as a sensing device for intertrial responses and time out. During the periods when the signal was presented, the switch could serve as a sensing device for defining a reinforced response.

DEVELOPING THE RESPONSE

Initially, a light under the response button was paired with the presentation of an auditory stimulus until stimulus control was achieved. The light then was faded (dimmed) until no light was visible. We found, as did Bricker and Bricker (1969), that the pairing of the response light and the auditory signal was not necessary. In fact, Bricker and Bricker indicated that this pairing increased training time. We currently use lights under the button (see Appendix B, Plate 4) for two purposes: (a) to light the response button continuously in order to assist the subject in isolating the button from the remainder of the response area, and (b) to indicate when the program is in effect; the light is connected to the program "on" switch.

Bringing the Response under Stimulus Control

In initial experiments, subjects were seated before the response-reinforcement apparatus. An auditory stimulus (500-Hz puretone) was presented (sound field). An experimenter attracted the subject's attention and demonstrated a response which resulted in the delivery of a reinforcer. It was necessary to direct the attention of some subjects to the reinforcer in the tray after the first two or three stimuli were presented.

During the next two or three trials, the experimenter placed the subject's hand on the response button. By this time, the subject usually attempted the response without assistance. If not, a nudge of his hand or arm was sufficient to complete a response. It is advisable for the experimenter to "fade" assistance to the subject as quickly as possible. If fading procedures are not effected, the touch and/or verbal prompt become the functional stimulus for a response. Patience and fading skills at this point are critical. Experimenters often maintain prompts too long and the subject simply does not respond until the prompt occurs. If an effective reinforcer has been established and no prompt is given, the subject usually learns to respond when no physical prompt is given. It is better to wait out the response than continually to assist the subject. Response development is usually the most difficult training phase for the subject and the most trying for the examiner's patience, yet most subjects can be trained to respond without assistance. The subject gradually becomes more and more proficient in responding, and responding comes under stimulus control.

Earphone Training

During the early phases of procedural development, training the subject to wear earphones followed developing a response and bringing it under auditory stimulus-response control. However, this was found to be an inefficient procedure. By initiating earphone training early, it is possible to delete all sound-field training procedures. The earphone-training phase, when necessary, now comes immediately after the selection of the reinforcement and before all other phases of the program. Most subjects readily accept earphones, and response development is initiated immediately.

When subjects resist the earphones, a training program is implemented in which the wearing of earphones becomes a discriminative stimulus for reinforcement. With persistent rejection of the earphones, it may be necessary to reintroduce them gradually. The subject is reinforced for allowing the earphones to be brought near. He then is required to allow them to be brought nearer and nearer until they are in place. As the subject learns to wear the earphones, the interval between reinforcers is lengthened systematically until the subject wears the phones for long periods of time without removing them. During the next phase, reinforcement is delivered for a response in the presence of the auditory stimulus. However, the auditory stimulus never is presented unless the subject is wearing the earphones. Reinforcement thus is contingent on two behaviors—wearing earphones and responding to the auditory signal.

Refining Response Development

At first, our subjects were trained to respond to the presence of a puretone and not to respond when the tone was absent. As our procedural research developed, we found that the presence/absence discrimination had serious consequences and limitations for tests such as the masked thresholds and the short-increment sensitivity index (SISI). Consequently, we decided to train the subjects to discriminate a *change in the auditory stimulus.* We trained subjects to respond to auditory changes (a) in a minimally audible environment (ambient noise), as found in threshold assessments, (b) in a noticeably audible background, as used in masked threshold procedures, and (c) in an auditory environment in which the background stimulus contains the same frequency properties as the discriminative stimulus itself, as found in the SISI. If a subject is trained to respond to the presentation of signals in the presence of a continuous noise, there is little difficulty in obtaining similar responses when the noise has been attenuated below threshold, as would be found in unmasked thresholds. Likewise, the subject already has been trained not to respond to mere background noise when obtaining masked thresholds. When the subject has been trained to detect stimulus change in a variety of auditory background situations, a variety of tests can be run with little additional training.

Response development is initiated with the binaural presence of a narrow-band (centered on 750 Hz) background stimulus [approximately 20 dB above the estimated threshold or 50 dB (hearing level)].

A 500-Hz signal, 5 seconds in duration, is used as the initial discriminative stimulus (S^D). The discriminative stimulus is presented at 40 dB above the estimated threshold or at 70-dB hearing level. With subjects suspected of having severe hearing losses, it may be necessary to increase the intensity of both the background (neutral) stimulus and the discriminative stimulus.

Once the subject has been trained to respond independently to the discriminative stimulus in the presence of a background stimulus, it is time to initiate a program to bring the response under even more precise stimulus control.

PROCEDURES FOR OBTAINING PRECISE STIMULUS CONTROL

Although the establishment of discriminative control begins immediately, the initial phases of the program concentrate on getting the subject to press the button. If the subject initially presses the button when the tone is absent, we do not become overly concerned. However, the subject must be under precise stimulus control prior to testing. This section details some of the problems associated with obtaining such precise control.

If a subject made a nondiscriminative response precisely at the moment of the onset of the discriminative stimulus, he was reinforced for an incorrect response even though he had not heard the stimulus. Likewise, if a subject responded simultaneously with the offset of the stimulus, no reinforcement occurred, resulting in a failure to reinforce a correct response. The probability that these two events will occur is low; however, they have happened. Such events have serious consequences early in a training program. To alleviate this problem, we inserted "predelay" and "postdelay" periods in the response circuit (see Figure 3). These periods are 300 milliseconds in duration. The stimulus must be present for at least 300 milliseconds in order to result in a reinforced response. The response circuit also remains open for 300 milliseconds after the termination of the signal; this accommodates a response at the end of the stimulus. In our experience, only one subject has responded

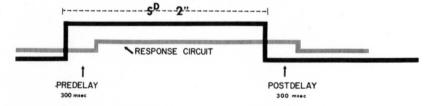

Figure 3. Graphic representation of stimulus, predelay, and postdelay relationships. (From Fulton and Spradlin, 1971.)

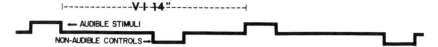

Figure 4. Graphic representation of audible stimulus and nonaudible control period relationships. (From Fulton and Spradlin, 1971.)

repeatedly between the onset of the stimulus and the opening of the response circuit (predelay period).

The postdelay period has important implications clinically or in subsequent short-stimulus-duration tests and experiments, used in later studies, i.e., SISI and psychoacoustics. The duration of the postdelay also can be lengthened by timer to accommodate a slow response of a cerebral palsied subject. However, the experimenter should remember that extensions of response time increase the possibility that random responses will be reinforced.

To evaluate whether a subject's responses are discriminative or random, control periods are inserted into the presentation program. With electromechanical relay equipment, the control periods alternate with discriminative stimuli (see Figure 4). With solid-state equipment, the discriminative stimuli and control periods are inserted by a probability generator. The control periods are nonaudible periods with the same temporal characteristics as those of the stimulus periods. Responses (button press) during the control periods have no consequences, but are recorded. To determine whether a subject is under stimulus control, responses during the discriminative stimulus period are compared with responses during the control periods. An example of a criterion we often use is illustrated in Figure 5. "Criterion" means responding to nine of 10 signal presentations and responding to no more than

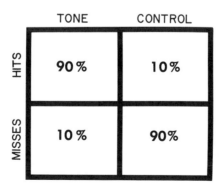

Figure 5. Example of stimulus control criteria. (From Fulton and Spradlin, 1971.)

one of 10 control periods, or, 9 S^D/1 control. A stimulus-response control criterion is established for each phase of training to ensure that each phase is learned before the experimenter proceeds to the next phase. Various criteria, established at the discretion of the experimenter, are used throughout these studies. Criterion levels have included 5/0 or 2/0 (responses to signal periods/ responses to control periods), both of which are 100 percent/0 percent.

There is some question as to whether the entire interval between signal presentations should be considered as the control period against which responses to the signals are compared. Such a measure would pose two problems. First, since responses occurring during the interval when the signal is not present delay the onset of the signal, the interval when the signal is not present is variable. Second, the subject can respond repeatedly when the signal is not present but he can respond only once to each signal.

Responses during either the discriminative stimulus or the control periods are recorded. They terminate that event and advance the program to the next event. If a response has not been made at the termination of that event, determined by timer, the program automatically advances to the next event.

The procedure presents an equal number of control and signal periods. The conditions required for presentation of both the signal and control periods are identical, and only one response is recorded for each period. This method allows evaluation of stimulus control by using simple probability statistics generated from the simple 2 × 2 table (see Figure 5).

The interval between events is termed the "intertrial interval" (ITI); it is determined by a tape programmer and can be programmed for any duration desired. To avoid temporal responding by the subject, the signal is presented on a variable interval (VI) schedule. Experience indicates that a VI-6 tape, i.e., variable, with a mean of 6 seconds, is effective. This schedule presents alternating stimulus and control events (as previously indicated, solid-state instrumentation uses a probability generator to determine the presentation order of stimulus and control periods) on a mean time interval of 6 seconds.

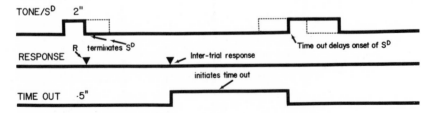

Figure 6. Graphic representation of stimulus, response, and time-out relationships. The dashed line indicates the program schedule had the subject not made a response. (From Fulton and Spradlin, 1971.)

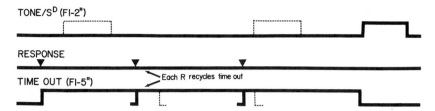

Figure 7. Graphic representation of effects of high-rate nondiscriminative responding. The dashed line indicates the program schedule had the subject not made a response. (From Fulton and Spradlin, 1971.)

This results in the discrimination signal's being presented on a VI schedule of 12 seconds plus the 2-second interval of the control period if no response occurs during the ITI.

Responses during the ITI are termed "intertrial responses" (ITR) and result in a 5-second time out, i.e., delay in the program, which precludes the presentation of the next event (a schematic of the stimulus, response, and time-out relationships is shown in Figure 6). High-rate ITR's result in minimal opportunity for subjects to be presented with discriminative stimuli, and hence minimal opportunity for reinforcement (see Figure 7). Each time an ITR is made, the time-out timer recycles noncumulatively.

Contact with the response area, previously discussed, also results in a time out for the duration of the contact plus the fixed time-out interval of 5 seconds.

During the initial response development training phase, the tone is presented for 5 seconds unless the subject responds before the 5-second limitation, in which case he is reinforced and the tone is terminated. This permits the subject ample time to respond to the signal. When the subject responds consistently within the 5-second period, the duration of the signal is reduced from 5 to 3 seconds and then to 2 seconds.

Generalization Procedures

Environmental Stimulus. To this point, training has concentrated on developing the desired response and bringing it under the control of a stimulus. The subject has been required to discriminate a 500-Hz discriminative stimulus in the presence of a 750-Hz, narrow-band background noise.

Next, the subject is trained to respond to the 500-Hz signal while the background condition is varied to include adjacent noise bands which are centered at 1 KHz and 500 Hz.

Upon meeting control criteria (see Appendix A) for noise-band generalization, the background noise is shifted to continuous background or pedestal puretone signals, 10 dB above the estimated threshold, in frequency orders of 1 KHz, 750 Hz, and 500 Hz. This order is a systematic shift from a background stimulus that differs from the discriminative stimulus to a condition in which the background and the discriminative stimuli are the same frequency. It is at this point that the response comes under the control of a change in the acoustic stimulus.

After discrimination has been achieved, the background stimulus is faded out, i.e., attenuated, to subthreshold levels. Experience indicates that once the subject has learned to respond under a variety of background conditions, a background stimulus can be inserted easily or withdrawn without loss of stimulus control. Hence the subject is trained for later masking or pedestal tone conditions.

Discriminative Stimulus Generalization. Now the subject is trained to respond to other frequencies in stimulus orders of .5 KHz, 1 KHz, 2 KHz, 4 KHz, 8 KHz, 2 KHz, and .25 KHz. Occasionally, a subject will not generalize readily across discriminative stimuli. A return to a previously successful frequency for two or three events and then back again usually will achieve generalization. On one or two occasions, it has been necessary to use interoctaves to achieve generalization. On only one occasion was it impossible to achieve generalization by the above procedure. In this case, it was necessary to return to the first phase for each frequency. The subject responded efficiently as he moved through the phases.

Intensity Generalization. By this time, the subject has been trained to respond to a clearly audible signal. It is important to make certain that the subject responds reliably to less intense signals. In this phase of training, the subject is required to respond to a 500-Hz signal as its intensity is reduced in 10-dB steps. This is continued until the subject quits responding or until normal sensitivity levels are reached. The procedure is repeated at 1 KHz. This phase may indicate possible hearing losses.

Unilateral generalization. Until now, all stimuli have been presented binaurally. The subject now is required to respond to the 500-Hz signal, 20–30 dB relative to estimated threshold, for each ear. Should this phase present a problem, it may indicate a unilateral loss.

The subject is now ready for audiometrical puretone screening or threshold assessment.

The principles[2] outlined in this chapter have far-reaching implications and hold true for a variety of difficult-to-test populations. These principles are

---

2 *Operant Audiometry with Retarded Children: Positive Reinforcement Discrimination,* a 16-mm color film, 16 minutes in duration, was produced in 1968 to demonstrate the basic principles for establishing stimulus-response control. This film illustrates method-

also basic for procedural application to a wide variety of auditory stimulus tasks; in fact, they hold for other sensory measurement tasks. In essence, the attainment of stimulus-response control is basic to this entire line of research and procedural application.

LITERATURE CITED

Bricker, D., and W. A. Bricker. 1969. A programmed approach to operant audiometry with low-functioning children. J. Speech Hear. Dis. 34: 312n 320.

Fulton, R. T. 1962. Psychogalvanic skin response and conditioned orientation reflex audiometry with mentally retarded children. Unpublished doctoral dissertation, Purdue University, Lafayette, Ind.

Fulton, R. T., and J. E. Spradlin. 1971. Operant audiometry with severely retarded children. Audiology 10: 203–211.

Hollis, J. H. 1973. "Superstition": The effects of independent and contingent events on free operant responses in retarded children. Am. J. Ment. Defic. 77: 585–596.

Liden, G., and A. Kankkunen. 1969. Visual reinforcement audiometry. Arch. Otolaryngol. 89: 865–872.

Lloyd, L. L. 1966. Behavioral audiometry viewed as an operant procedure. J. Speech Hear. Dis. 31: 128–136.

Nowles, M. M. 1971. Operant audiometry with two year olds. Unpublished master's thesis, Kansas State University, Manhattan, Kan.

Spradlin, J. E., and L. L. Lloyd. 1965. Operant conditioning audiometry (OCA) with low level retardates: A preliminary report. In: L. L. Lloyd and D. R. Frisina (eds.), The Audiologic Assessment of the Mentally Retarded: Proceedings of a National Conference, pp. 45–58. Parsons State Hospital and Training Center, Parsons, Kan.

Spradlin, J. E., L. L. Lloyd, G. L. Hom, and M. J. Reid. 1968. Establishing tone control and evaluating the hearing of severely retarded children. In: G. A. Jervis (ed.), Expanding Concepts in Mental Retardation, pp. 170–180. Charles C Thomas, Springfield, Ill.

Suzuki, T., and Y. Ogiba. 1960. A technique of puretone audiometry for children under three years of age: Conditioned orientation reflex (C.O.R.) audiometry. Rev. Laryngol. 1: 33–45.

Suzuki, T., and Y. Ogiba. 1961. Conditioned orientation reflex audiometry. Arch. Otolaryngol. 74: 192–198.

---

ology used in the early stages of developing this procedure and therefore differs somewhat from the above description of a training procedure. However, many of the basic principles are similar. A subsequent 16-mm color film, 9 minutes in duration, called *The Temporal Parameters of Auditory Stimulus-Response Control* and produced in 1973, illustrates and discusses the programming elements of the procedure as discussed in the text. Both films are available through the Audio-Visual Center, 6 Bailey Hall, University of Kansas, Lawrence, Kansas 66045 for nominal handling costs.

2 Evaluation of Stimulus-Response Control Training Procedures

Robert T. Fulton

The efficiency of the 10-phase stimulus-response control training procedures discussed in Chapter 1 and specified in Appendix A was evaluated with 50 untrained, difficult-to-test, severely retarded children and adolescents. The subjects (15 females, 35 males) ranged in age from 7 years, 8 months to 19 years, 1 month, with a mean of 11 years, 8 months. Their Intelligence (IQ) or Social Quotients (SQ) ranged from a low of 12 to a high of 68 (high was a deaf child), with a mean of 31.9. All subjects were considered difficult-to-test, i.e., unresponsive to standard handraising audiometric procedures, and were unfamiliar with operant audiometric training procedures.

The training procedures were administered prior to initial operant audiometric intake procedures in a residential institution for the retarded. The 10-phase training procedure specified in Appendix A was used with all subjects. In addition, all subjects were required to meet each individual phase criterion before advancing to the next phase. The subsequent audiometric assessment varied from puretone screening to complete masked thresholds, including bone-conduction thresholds. One subject was found to be deaf.

Electromechanical programming instrumentation (see Appendix C, Plate 1) and a standard two-channel audiometer were used to control the stimulus, response, and consequence events.

Electromechanical counters recorded the number of stimulus presentations, control periods, responses to stimuli, responses during control periods, and total responses. A clock attached to the program switch indicated the duration of each phase in seconds. Data were recorded for each subject for each phase of the training procedure.

The data were evaluated to determine the number of stimulus presentations, the number of responses to stimuli, and the test time required to meet the criterion for each phase. The total number of responses made also was recorded. An abbreviated illustration of results may be found in Table 1. The group and raw data indicate:

1. The median training time required to train and prepare difficult-to-test subjects to respond to audiometric test procedures was 1 hour, 35 minutes. In view of the fact that two or three subjects indicated high training times, the median appeared to be a better indicator of test times than the mean.

2. The difficulty experienced by subjects was not consistent across phases. For instance, the subject who indicated the longest training time for Phase 3 indicated the shortest time for Phase 4, was above the mean time for Phase 5, and below the mean time for Phase 6. It appears that some subjects are affected by variables other than the program or procedure. For example, a subject temporarily may not be under good reinforcement control because of satiation, illness, emotional state, etc., yet he may fall under good control again after these conditions subside.

3. In every phase, at least one subject was able to meet the criterion in the minimal number of trials. The mean number of trials required by the subjects to meet criteria in relation to the minimal number of procedural trials required to meet criteria was reasonably constant, i.e., there was high individual subject variability between phases, yet group mean consistency between phases. This suggested that the degree of difficulty for each training phase was relatively constant. However, that is not to say that the procedures are not subject to improvement.

TRAINING WITH REDUCED CRITERIA

Three additional subjects were brought under good stimulus control in fewer trials (reduced response criteria). Although the data are not included and these subjects were not included in the above evaluation, it was demonstrated that the stringent criteria established for completion of each phase were not necessary for all subjects. They were required to complete the 10-phase training program as written, except that the 5 S^D/0 control response criterion was reduced to 3 and 0. These subjects, ranging in age from 9 to 20 years and in IQ from 35 to 68, met training criteria in a mean time of 31 minutes, 40 seconds. Not all subjects should be or can be adequately trained by an abbreviated procedure; however, it is applicable in many instances without sacrificing stimulus control.

Table 1. Condensed table of stimulus presentations, stimulus responses, total responses, and test times per phase of the stimulus-response control, audiometrical pretest training program (See Appendix A for procedural details)

Training phase	Minimal no. of presentations required to meet criteria	$\bar{X}$ Stimulus presentations	$\bar{X}$ Stimulus responses	$\bar{X}$ Total responses	Test time (hr/min/sec) Mean	Median
1	Variable	91.5	55.5	205.4	−/38/55	−/11/20
2	5	17.8	13.6	47.4	−/ 9/22	−/ 3/20
3	5	19.4	11.1	30.4	−/ 7/57	−/ 3/ 0
4	5	20.0	12.3	41.6	−/ 8/ 1	−/ 2/32
5	10	30.0	18.1	62.6	−/12/33	−/ 6/15
6	15	39.1	25.8	80.5	−/15/16	−/ 7/56
7	8	18.4	14.2	31.7	−/ 6/52	−/ 4/28
8	16	30.0	20.4	43.0	−/10/55	−/ 7/10
9	10	25.7	17.9	40.8	−/ 9/31	−/ 8/16
10	10	19.8	13.8	28.7	−/ 8/ 6	−/ 4/52
Total	84+	311.7*	202.7*	612.1*	2/ 7/48	1/35/36

*Total of means.

A less stringent training criterion might reduce the time required to train subjects to the point of threshold measurement. However, short-cutting the training procedure may lead to less reliable results or to the necessity for additional training for other tests. If testing beyond screening is not required, some training phases may be reduced or eliminated. The recommended program (Appendix A) has been designed for maximal utility and generalization across test procedures.

CARRY-OVER

Clinical experience indicates that once a subject has completed the response training program, subsequent retraining programs require much less effort. Subjects who have not been confronted with the operant audiometric procedure for periods as long as 4 years have demonstrated they can respond appropriately within six S^D presentations (reevaluation) without assistance.

Reid (1969), studying the effects of reinforcement on stimulus control and thresholds, used subjects who had been evaluated initially by operant procedures 2 years before his investigation. His subjects were chosen on the clinical assumption that retraining procedures could be hastened and because the training phases were not a critical area of investigation. Records of the eight severely retarded children (measured intelligence levels IV and V) showed that a mean of 264.7 stimulus presentations were necessary to meet initial training criteria. Phase or session times were not recorded for the initial training sessions.

Two years later, the same subjects required an average of 178.6 stimulus presentations to meet Reid's training criteria. The mean pretraining time required was 87.45 minutes. Four of the subjects met Reid's criteria in less than 60 minutes. One subject required 389 minutes. Because of continual programming development, the same procedure was not used in both instances, but it does suggest that some degree of training retention was evident, or that the procedures had been improved between the first and second training programs.

Clinical records of six severely retarded children who had not been reevaluated for approximately 4 years required an average of 193 stimulus presentations and 1 hour and 16 minutes to meet retraining criteria. Again, it should be noted that a minimum of 90 presentations are required to meet all training phase criteria in the recommended program.

Four severely retarded subjects, ranging in age from 12 years, 7 months to 15 years, 7 months, who had not had contact with the operant puretone procedure for over 2 years (range of 2 years, 3 months to 5 years, 2 months) were selected as subjects in an applied research project. Their performance on the 10-phase training schedule indicated that they were able to meet training criteria with a mean training time of 40 minutes, 56 seconds, using a mean number of 122 stimulus presentations.

These examples of subject groups suggest that retraining requires less time than does the initial training time.

UNSUCCESSFUL ATTEMPTS AT TRAINING

During the period of the training program evaluation for the 50 severely retarded children, four severely retarded children were encountered for whom the procedure was unsuccessful.

Case P. T. Age 10 years, 5 months. The subject had poor vision and ambulation and could not feed herself. She had no apparent awareness of the tone and never pushed the button independently. After 6 hours, 5 minutes, 50 seconds (15 sessions), the subject had not met criteria for Phase 1 and was excused.

Case C. E. Age 8 years, 5 months. The subject completed the first three phases in 20 minutes, 40 seconds. Halfway into the second session, the subject quit responding. Conditioning was still unsuccessful when breakfast was withheld in an attempt to strengthen the reinforcer. Response could not be reestablished after an additional 2 hours, 4 minutes, 40 seconds (eight sessions) of training time.

Case G. H. Age 13 years, 10 months. The subject met the 10-phase training criteria after 6 hours, 38 minutes (23 sessions) of training, but after an additional 2 hours, 17 minutes, 42 seconds (10 sessions), the subject did not meet criteria for assessing threshold or screening. Even after breakfast was withheld, conditioning was unsuccessful.

Case D. B. Age 7 years, 8 months. Two hours, 42 minutes, 40 seconds (seven sessions) were required to train the subject to wear earphones. After an additional 1 hour, 58 minutes (five sessions), the subject had not met the criterion for Phase 1 of the training program. This child spent most of the time kicking and screaming. Although some improvement was noted in her behavior, it was insufficient to warrant continued training attempts.

The procedure was not successful for these four cases; however, the ratio of successful/unsuccessful attempts (50 and four, respectively) is highly encouraging because all of the subjects were termed difficult-to-test, having demonstrated nonresponsiveness to standard handraising procedures. The four unsuccessful cases were representative of the type of problems found clinically: lack of appropriate reinforcement, incompatible behavior, and gross motor problems.

SUMMARY

The research reported in this chapter demonstrates that if the principles of behavioral control are applied in a systematic manner, most severely handicapped children can be taught the discrimination response necessary for auditory evaluation. The precise and systematic application of behavioral procedures was achieved through the use of instrumentation. As Lloyd (1966) has indicated, many of the principles can be used without complicated instrumentation. Nevertheless, instrumentation allows for a degree of precision which cannot be obtained otherwise. In addition, it is more feasible to replicate what a machine does than what a clinician does. For these reasons, we have relied heavily on programming instrumentation throughout our research efforts.

LITERATURE CITED

Lloyd, L. L. 1966. Behavioral audiometry viewed as an operant procedure. J. Speech Hear. Dis. 31: 128–136.

Reid, M. J. 1969. Effects of reinforcement on auditory stimulus control and threshold assessment with retarded children. Unpublished master's thesis, Kansas State University, Manhattan, Kan.

Applications to Audiometric Technology

The preceding chapters discussed the principles and procedures required to obtain basic auditory stimulus-response control with difficult-to-test persons. Yet those procedures are not an end in themselves. With the model proposed, the attainment of basic auditory discriminative response is a necessary requirement, but it does not provide the measures necessary to complete an appropriate audiologic diagnosis.

It is doubtful that many clinicians would advocate audiologic diagnosis based on puretone threshold measurements alone. However, an audiologic test battery probably would receive unanimous support. Therefore, the question is not whether we should have test batteries, but how such an assessment battery can be achieved with difficult-to-test populations.

Such a goal requires precise behavioral control procedures as well as procedures which control and present stimuli with specified parameters.

This section presents three procedural applications: puretone thresholds, the short-increment sensitivity index (SISI), and threshold tone decay. This does not mean that the test battery should be limited to these three procedures or that they are the most important, nor does it mean that they are not subject to improvement. However, the procedures are representative of peripheral, cochlear, and retrocochlear problems and they easily are adaptable to the proposed model.

Each procedure is presented individually with appropriate cross-referencing, and each is based on the premise that behavioral, i.e., stimulus-response, control is a basic interprocedural prerequisite.

3 Puretone Threshold Measurement

Robert T. Fulton and
Joseph E. Spradlin

One of the major criteria of any clinical procedure is that it produce reliable findings. The three studies of this chapter address this issue directly. The first study evaluates test-retest thresholds obtained by ascending-descending procedures; the second evaluates the reliability of thresholds obtained by a different control criterion; and the third experiment evaluates the effect of continuous and intermittent reinforcement on threshold measures.

RELIABILITY

Our puretone threshold measurement experiments initially attempted to answer two questions: (a) do operant audiometric procedures yield reliable (intersession) threshold measures? and (b) do ascending and descending measurement techniques result in similar threshold values?

In our first experiment (Spradlin, Locke, and Fulton, 1969), the subjects were six severely retarded children (IQ-SQ range 20–45, X = 28.5) ranging in chronologic age from 8 years, 8 months to 16 years, 10 months ($\overline{X}$ = 12 years, 2 months). The preexperimental training procedures and instrumentation described in Chapter 1 were used. Prior to the initial experimental session, a clinically estimated threshold (1 KHz) was obtained by operant procedures for each subject for the test ear. The estimated threshold (ET) did not follow a specified procedure but was judged subjectively to be representative of the subject's threshold.

Prior to each experimental threshold measurement, the subject was required to meet stimulus-response control criteria by responding to nine of 10 consecutive stimuli (20 dB above ET) while responding to no more than one of 10 intervening control periods.

Thresholds were obtained during six experimental sessions. Descending-ascending techniques were counterbalanced between sessions. A descending schedule consisted of an auditory stimulus of 1 KHz presented at 10 dB above the ET, followed by a control period, with alternating (stimulus/control) intervals presented in descending 5-dB increments to a point 10 dB below the ET [+10, control (C), +5, C, ET, C, −5, C, −10, C]. The ascending schedule followed the same format, beginning at 10 dB below the ET, and ascending and descending stimulus series were presented five times in each session for a total of 25 stimuli per session. The session threshold was defined as the lowest intensity at which the subject responded to at least three of five presentations for a given intensity.

Variances in threshold measures are found in Figure 1. In no instance did thresholds exceed a 15-dB range, and in at least five of six measures for each subject, thresholds were within a ± 5-dB range. Results indicate good inter-session consistency of operant threshold procedures with severely retarded children. Five of the six subjects indicated threshold patterns slightly above the ET, suggesting that strict threshold criteria yield slightly higher thresholds than subjective evaluations (ET). There was no pattern of ascending-descending technique effects.

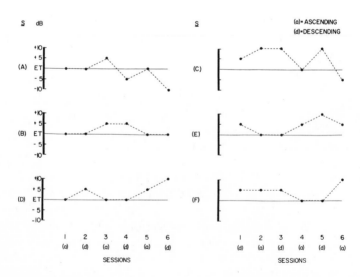

Figure 1. Session-threshold variances around the estimated threshold (*ET*) for each subject using ascending (*a*) and descending (*d*) techniques. $\underline{S}$, subject. (From Spradlin et al., 1969.)

The ascending-descending techniques used in the above experiment did not follow the procedures established by Hughson and Westlake (1944) and Carhart and Jerger (1959), respectively. In both of these procedures, the respective stimulus presentation pattern is recycled as soon as the subject responds (ascending) or fails to respond (descending). In this experiment, the presentation schedule continued until five stimuli had been presented before recycling. Each subject was presented with an equal number of trials. With either of the two traditional techniques, the number of trials differs between subjects and between sessions.

As implied by Lloyd (1966), there is a certain logical inference which can be made to support the descending technique (Carhart and Jerger, 1959) when reinforcement procedures are used. When a subject is reinforced for each correct response, there is multiple opportunity for reinforcement with each descending series of trials. There is an opportunity for only one reinforced response with each ascending series (Hughson and West-lake, 1944). Also, ascending techniques require what appear perceptually to the subject to be longer intervals between trials than do the descending techniques, based on the fact that trials between stimulus identi-fication responses are subthreshold.

Our second experiment (Fulton and Spradlin, 1971) attempted to exam-ine further the factors of ascending-descending measurement techniques and stimulus-response control. The purposes of this experiment were (a) to exam-ine threshold variability in relation to traditional ascending (Carhart and Jerger, 1959) and descending (Hughson and Westlake, 1944) measurement techniques, and (b) to examine the effects of different stimulus-control criteria on threshold measurement.

This experiment used three groups of six subjects each. All subjects were severely retarded. Group A met the stimulus-response control criteria before initiation of each test session. Group B met the criteria only once, on the day before the experimental sessions began. Group C was not required to meet any criteria, but was required to be familiar with the procedure.

The subjects ranged in chronological age from 8 years, 2 months to 20 years, 1 month, and in intelligence or social quotients from 13 to 45. There was no relationship among age, intelligence, and group assignment.

Ascending and descending schedules, alternating between sessions, were administered in the traditional way as described by Hughson and Westlake and by Carhart and Jerger. That is, rather than presenting an equal number of trials, as in the first experiment, the schedules were recycled for an appropri-ate response on the ascending schedule or a "miss" for the descending schedule. In this experiment, subjects had the opportunity for multiple reinforcement in each descending schedule cycle, one for each correct response. They had only one opportunity for reinforcement in each ascending schedule cycle.

As in the previous experiment, a clinically estimated threshold (1 KHz, test ear) was obtained for each subject before the actual experimental sessions were begun. Experimental thresholds for both schedules were defined as the lowest intensity level at which a 50-percent response rate was maintained for at least six trials, while less than a 50-percent response rate for six trials was maintained at the next lower intensity level.

Group A, which met daily control criteria, yielded the least variable threshold measurements. Five of the six subjects indicated test-retest consistency of ± 5 dB or less (see Figure 2). The sixth subject provided thresholds within a 15-dB range or less.

Subjects A5 and A6 differed from the estimated threshold but demonstrated intrasubject consistency. This suggests that the subjects were internally consistent and that the estimated threshold was judged to be better than experimental thresholds obtained by the 50-percent criterion used in this experiment.

Group B, which met the criteria only once before the initial experimental session, indicated slightly greater threshold variability than Group A (see Figure 3). Five of the six subjects indicated thresholds within a 10-dB range for at least five of the six sessions. Subject B5 indicated a bizarre threshold on the fifth session. In clinical testing, this type of behavior is noted when stimulus-response control criteria are not used. This is to say that, often for some unknown reason, subjects do not provide appropriate responses on any given day. These responses can be spotted by the application of a stimulus-response control criterion; thus, thresholds are not measured for that day.

Group C, which was not required to meet any control criteria, yielded the greatest variability between threshold measures (see Figure 4).

Overall variability effects by groups suggested that establishment of stimulus control criteria is the major effect.

We thought that if stimulus-response control were a major variable and if the various stimulus-response control criteria used were feasible indices of that control, threshold variability could be reduced by the application of the more stringent daily criteria. Therefore, four subjects from Groups B and C indicating the greatest variability were reevaluated by a daily stimulus-response control criterion.

Figure 5 indicates that the variability between thresholds was reduced for two of these subjects. One subject, C2, who previously had been cooperative but variable in his threshold responses, refused to respond to any stimuli for any test session. Apparently, the reinforcing agent used with C2 no longer maintained its reinforcing properties. Subject C1 responded consistently,

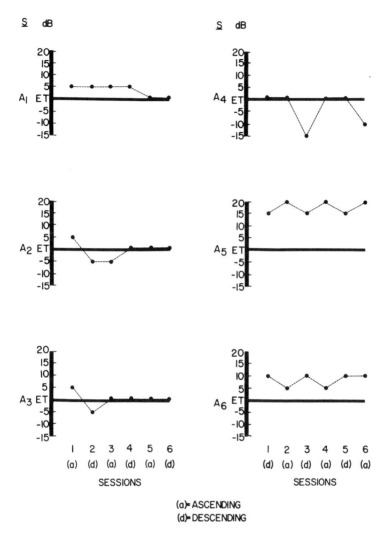

Figure 2. Ascending-descending thresholds (1 KHz) obtained for each subject in Group A for each of six sessions. Subjects were required to meet stimulus control criteria prior to each session (*ET,* estimated threshold; S subject). (From Fulton and Spradlin, 1971.)

within ± 10 dB, until the last session. No explanation for this behavior can be given other than that occasionally a subject meets stimulus-response control criteria at the beginning of a session, yet loses control later in the session. In this case, it was apparent that aberrant behavior was occurring

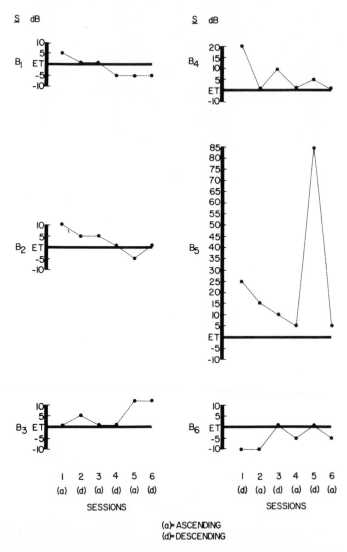

Figure 3. Ascending-descending thresholds (1 KHz) obtained for each subject in Group B for each of six sessions. Subjects were required to meet stimulus control criteria once on the day prior to the initial experimental session (*ET*, estimated threshold; $\underline{S}$, subject). (From Fulton and Spradlin, 1971.)

before threshold was fully determined. Clinically, modification would be made to bring the subject back to appropriate levels; otherwise, he would be excused for the day. In our experiment, we used "by-the-book" applications. Thus, all subjects were treated equally. Three of the four subjects demonstrated consistency within a 15-dB range for at least five of the six sessions. Two of the subjects did not exceed a 10-dB range.

Ascending-descending techniques and their respective reinforcement schedules were not a critical variable for any of the groups. The results

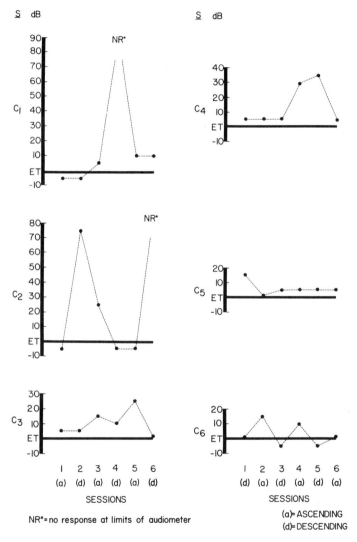

Figure 4. Ascending-descending threshold (1 KHz) obtained for each subject in Group C for each of six sessions. Subjects were not required to meet stimulus control criteria, but were required to be familiar with the test procedure (*ET*, estimated threshold; S, subject). (From Fulton and Spradlin, 1971.)

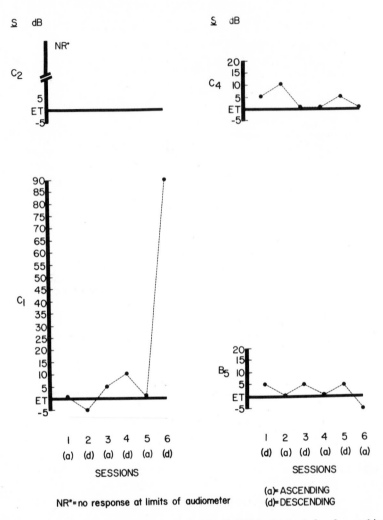

Figure 5. Ascending and descending thresholds (1 KHz) obtained for four subjects (Groups B and C) indicating prior high threshold variability when stimulus control was required prior to each experimental session (*ET*, estimated threshold; S, subject). (From Fulton and Spradlin, 1971.)

suggest that stimulus-response control is a major variable. The results of these experiments suggest that reliable audiograms can be obtained from severely retarded children with the operant procedures described.

Effects of Reinforcement on Reliability

Thus far, little has been said about the effects of reinforcement schedules on threshold assessment and reliability. Partial reinforcement is more resistant to extinction than is continuous reinforcement, but proper use of partial reinforcement usually requires that the subject be trained to accept it. Because audiometric assessments usually do not require long-term evaluation, it does not seem advantageous to impose a partial reinforcement training program. Satiation usually can be handled by not extending sessions to a point at which the reinforcer becomes ineffective. Also, reinforcer variability minimizes satiation effects.

In an informal experiment, the effects of reinforcement on thresholds were evaluated. In conjunction with the investigation by Reid (1969), the present investigators independently assessed threshold variability of six of Reid's eight subjects under continuous (CRF) and fixed ratio (FR-3) reinforcement schedules. All subjects (mean age, 10 years, 6 months) were severely retarded and indicated measured intelligence levels of IV or V (Heber, 1961). No program to train acceptance of partial reinforcement was initiated. Subjects were required to meet stimulus-response control criteria, i.e., to respond to nine of 10 stimuli and to no more than one of 10 control periods for 10 consecutive pairs of stimuli, prior to each threshold assessment. Continuous reinforcement schedules provided reinforcement for each correct response, whereas fixed ratio (FR-3) schedules reinforced each third correct response. Descending measurement techniques were used. Threshold was defined as the lowest intensity at which a 50-percent response rate could be maintained for at least six stimulus trials.

Threshold variability, by reinforcement schedule, is indicated in Figure 6. No apparent differences were noted between CRF and FR-3 thresholds. In only one session did a subject (J. H.) indicate a variability of 15 dB from the central tendency. These results add strength to previous data which indicated that operant thresholds with severely retarded children provide intersession consistency. This was particularly true with K. D., who indicated ± 5-dB consistency over 32 sessions.

A portion of Reid's study was directed toward nonreinforced threshold assessment subsequent to maintenance periods of reinforced (CRF and FR-3) stimulus discriminations. In this study, two groups of four severely retarded children each were used as subjects. The two groups were in a counterbalance design, as shown in Table 1. Pretraining procedures followed the method of Hughson and Westlake, with a maximum of 50 trials for each threshold session. "Threshold" was defined as the lowest intensity level at which a

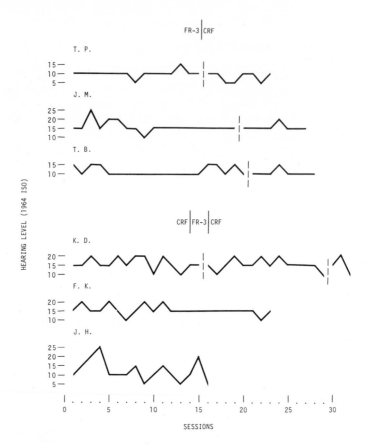

Figure 6. Threshold variability (1 KHz) of subject assessed by continuous (*CRF*) and fixed ratio (*FR-3*) reinforcement schedules.

minimum of four stimulus presentations were presented and correctly identified 50 percent of the time. Responses during the threshold session were not reinforced.

Results indicated that four subjects (two from each group) provided thresholds at all four measurement sessions within ± 5-dB variability. Two subjects failed to meet the threshold criterion in the first session; however, subsequent sessions provided threshold variability of 10 dB or less. The remaining two subjects indicated highly variable thresholds or did not meet the criteria. The results were favorable in view of the fact that thresholds were measured under conditions of extinction, i.e., with no reinforcement. The latter two subjects did not respond well even under reinforced (either CRF or FR-3) conditions of stimulus discrimination, thus suggesting ineffec-

Table 1. Counterbalance design for subject groups

	4 Sessions	1 Session	4 Sessions	1 Session	4 Sessions	1 Session
Group A						
Condition*	Stimulus control	Threshold assessment	Stimulus control	Threshold assessment	Stimulus control	Threshold assessment
Reinforcement†	CRF	None	FR-3	None	CRF	None
Group B						
Condition	Stimulus control	Threshold assessment	Stimulus control	Threshold assessment	Stimulus control	Threshold assessment
Reinforcement	FR-3	None	CRF	None	FR-3	None

*Stimulus control = stimulus control maintenance, 15 dB re: estimated threshold. Threshold assessment = auditory threshold assessment, Hughson-Westlake descending technique.
†CRF, continuous reinforcement; FR-3, fixed ratio reinforcement; None, no reinforcement.
(From Reid, 1969.)

tive reinforcement. Although no formal analysis was made, Reid found that three distinct patterns were in evidence when the lowest intensity response to each descending series was plotted. One pattern indicated no extinction over time. The second indicated stability for approximately half of the series; then extinction effects became apparent. In the last, extinction became effective almost immediately, resulting in a 90-dB shift by the end of the session.

There was no clear-cut distinction between thresholds preceded by either CRF or FR-3 auditory discrimination sessions. It appeared that stimulus-response control was a greater factor than reinforcement schedules.

Both of the above schedules are forms of fixed reinforcement schedules. The CRF schedule is actually a FR-1. In view of reinforcement schedules used in other behavioral tasks, it seems likely that an intermittent schedule on a variable ratio would increase resistance to extinction.

Reliability with Other Populations

Nowles (1971), using a procedure modified from that described, investigated test-retest consistency with 10 normal 2-year-olds (age range, 18–30 months; mean age, 26.3 months). Test-retest thresholds were obtained at three frequencies (250 Hz, 1 KHz, and 4 KHz) for the test ear. Results indicated that 25 of the 30 test-retest threshold comparisons (83 percent) yielded no differences, and the remaining five were within ± 5 dB. All but one subject indicated thresholds within the normal range. Results indicate that operant procedures are applicable and reliable in work with young children.

Although we have not completed formal investigations with infant populations, we have successfully on many occasions used these procedures in clinical practice and have found them successful to the age of 12 months. Lloyd, Spradlin, and Reid (1968) reported successful clinical threshold measurements of children as young as 7 months.

Reliability investigations of operant bone-conduction thresholds have not been completed, but there is no reason to suspect that similar results would not be obtained, inasmuch as the only variables are in sound transmission or transducer placement.

VALIDITY

Once the question of reliability has been answered, validity becomes the key question. To state that reliable measures are valid ignores the possibility that they are consistently suprathreshold. This is true whether one is using operant or any other procedures. One method of establishing validity is through a demonstration of a unilateral sensorineural loss. This shows that responses are related to unilateral and frequency differences; thus, it is unlikely that the subject has resorted to a suprathreshold internal reference. This same deductive procedure is applicable to children with conductive losses where bone-conduction responses are at or near zero-intensity levels. During 7 years of clinical testing, examples have occurred in sufficient numbers (most verified through medical referral) that validity has been assumed when stimulus-response control, procedural control, and threshold rechecking procedures have been followed.

Ghiselli (1964) states:

> Sometimes validity refers to the degree to which a set of operations measures the traits it is supposed to measure, and sometimes it refers to the determination of the traits actually measured by a set of operations. . . . Whereas we say that with reliability of measurement it is possible to formulate different definitions in reasonably precise ways, this is not always the case with validity of measurement.

In the first two experiments, both ascending and descending threshold methodologies were used. The purposes discussed and implied were related to the effects of methodology on threshold values. The question, at the time of the experiment, was keyed to the effects of the methodology. However, those same data can be used to define validity. If one assumes that a descending methodology is a standard referent (independent methodology), then the ascending procedure becomes the dependent methodology. One then can assume concurrent or predictive validity between the two procedures. Specifically, one can predict the same values for the ascending methodology, given the values for the descending procedure.

The principles underlying the errors of *habituation* (tendency to continue to report "yes" in a descending series), and *anticipation* (report "no" in an ascending series), the instrumental control of $S \rightarrow R$ relationships, and the convergence of methodology strongly support the premise that the trait, i.e., the threshold, has been measured validly. These conditions control for the establishment of supra- or subthreshold referents. Convergence then may be considered the measure of response validity, and the data indicate that the converging methodologies provided similar threshold values.

CLINICAL APPLICATION

The results of our experiments and clinical experience in measuring puretone thresholds have led us to adopt the following clinical procedures, which we have found to be successful. We do feel, however, that once a subject has been trained to the criteria of stimulus-response control, any of several screening and threshold measurement procedures are applicable (also see Appendix A, Phase 2.)

Screening

Subjects are required to meet a stimulus-response control criterion, i.e., to respond to nine stimuli with no more than one response to a control period for 10 consecutive pairs of events, at the beginning of each session before screening measurements are begun. Measurements are repeated to check for consistency.

Thresholds

Subjects are required to meet the stimulus-response control criterion at the beginning of each threshold assessment session. The Hughson-Westlake descending procedure is used. "Threshold" is defined as the lowest intensity at which the subject maintains a 50-percent response rate for a minimum of six trials. Bone-conduction thresholds are determined in the same manner as air-conduction thresholds.

Masking procedures are applied routinely in accordance with masking rules established by Studebaker (1964) regarding air-conduction:

Mask the ear opposite the tested ear whenever the air-conduction threshold of the tested ear exceeds the bone-conduction threshold of the masked ear by 35 to 50 dB (35 dB at low frequencies, 40 to 45 dB at speech frequencies, and 50 dB at high frequencies).

and bone-conduction:

Always apply a masking noise to the opposite ear when testing the bone-conduction threshold of an ear with an air-bone gap of ten dB or more.

(The use of Studebaker's procedures should not become a procedural issue of debate with other well-supported procedures. It is offered only as a procedure which has been used clinically. A theoretical debate of masking procedures is not the purpose of this chapter.)

Masking Training Procedures Preceding Assessment

Subjects were introduced to masking principles in the stimulus-response control training phase; therefore, when masking procedures are required, it is necessary to reintroduce the masking stimulus only briefly. This is done in a three-phase procedure (see Appendix A, Phases 12–14).

Phase 12. Present 500-Hz discriminative stimulus (S^D) (2 seconds) binaurally at 30-dB sensation level (SL), for the better ear, with narrow-band

(500-Hz) masking at 30-dB SL [masking is calibrated with filters (Allison 22; Tracor, Medical Instruments Division, Austin, Tex.) in "out" position]. Present stimuli until subject meets a 5 S^D/0 control criterion (see discussion of criteria in Chapter 1).

Phase 13. Increase masking level by 10 dB. Present stimuli until subject meets 5/0 criterion.

Phase 14. Generalize to other frequencies (1 KHz, 2 KHz, 4 KHz, 250 Hz) with accompanying masking at 20 dB below S^D, S^D at 30 dB SL. To meet the criterion, the subject must make 2/0 consecutive responses for each frequency before moving to the next frequency. If the subject misses two consecutive responses, the examiner should return to the previously successful frequency. When the subject has met the criteria, he is ready for masked threshold assessment.

SUMMARY

Evidence was provided to indicate that operant procedures provide effective, reliable, and substantially valid methods for assessing puretone thresholds with retarded children. There is also empirical evidence to indicate that these procedures are applicable to a wide variety of difficult-to-test populations.

The maintenance of stimulus-response control appears to be a more critical factor than the choice of threshold searching techniques (ascending-descending) or reinforcement schedules.

LITERATURE CITED

Carhart, R., and J. F. Jerger. 1959. Preferred method for clinical determination of puretone thresholds. J. Speech Hear. Dis. 24: 330–345.

Fulton, R. T., and J. E. Spradlin. 1971. Operant audiometry with severely retarded children. Audiology 10: 203–211.

Ghiselli, E. E. 1964. Theory of Psychological Measurement. McGraw-Hill, New York.

Heber, R. 1961. Measured intelligence: A manual on terminology and classification in mental retardation. Amer. J. Ment. Defic. (Monogr. Suppl.) 64: 57–60.

Hughson, W., and H. Westlake. 1944. Manual for program outline for rehabilitation of aural casualties both military and civilian. Trans. Amer. Acad. Ophthalmol. Otolaryngol. (Suppl.) 48: 1–15.

Lloyd, L. L. 1966. Behavioral audiometry viewed as an operant procedure. J. Speech Hear. Dis. 31: 128–136.

Lloyd, L. L., J. E. Spradlin, and M. J. Reid. 1968. An operant audiometric procedure for difficult-to-test patients. J. Speech Hear. Dis. 33: 236–245.

Nowles, M. M. 1971. Operant audiometry with two year olds. Unpublished master's thesis, Kansas State University, Manhattan, Kan.

Reid, M. J. 1969. Effects of reinforcement on auditory stimulus control and threshold assessment with retarded children. Unpublished master's thesis, Kansas State University, Manhattan, Kan.

Spradlin, J. E., B. J. Locke, and R. T. Fulton. 1969. Conditioning and audiological assessment. *In*: R. T. Fulton and L. L. Lloyd (eds.), Audiometry for the Retarded: With Implications for the Difficult-to-Test, pp. 125–163. Williams & Wilkins, Baltimore.

Studebaker, G. A. 1964. Clinical masking of air- and bone-conducted stimuli. J. Speech Hear. Dis. 29: 23–35.

4 The Short-Increment Sensitivity Index

Robert T. Fulton and
Joseph E. Spradlin

Because the stimulus-response control procedures had been effective in evaluating puretone thresholds, it was assumed that they also might be useful in obtaining other audiologic information from severely retarded children. The short-increment sensitivity index (SISI) seemed adaptable to operant techniques. The SISI, a test of the ability of a subject to detect small-intensity differences of short duration, assists the audiologist in differentiating cochlear pathologies from other auditory conditions and from normal ears (Harford, 1967; Jerger, 1962a, b; Jerger, Shedd, and Harford, 1959; Martin, 1972). The SISI uses a puretone stimulus, as do conventional threshold measurements; however, it differs in temporal and intensity characteristics. It requires the subject to detect intensity changes by increments in a continuous puretone pedestal signal, usually presented at 20 dB SL. The ability of a subject to detect a high percentage (60–100 percent) of 1-dB intensity changes is considered a positive finding and is associated with cochlear dysfunction. Inability to detect more than 20 percent of the signals is considered a negative finding. The ability to identify 25–55 percent of the stimuli is considered a questionable finding.

An experiment was effected to investigate the development of SISI procedures and to assess their applicability with the severely retarded. The basic instrumentation and programming parameters were similar to those of previous experiments. Only procedural modifications as described within the experiment were required.

INSTRUMENTATION

Auditory stimuli, i.e., signal intensity increments and pedestal tone, were generated and controlled by an Allison 22 audiometer and fed to TDH-39

earphones with MX-41/AR cushions. The audiometer was calibrated periodically. All pretraining and test procedures were conducted in a noise-
controlled environment (Industrial Acoustics Co., Bronx, N. Y.). The same
programming schematic as that used with puretone threshold was used with
the SISI (see Appendix C, Plate 1).

For experimental procedures, the optical interceptor board (SISI adapter)
of the Allison 22 was replaced with a modified board (Appendix C, Plate 2)
which was activated by the programming apparatus, rather than by the
standard photocell trigger. Photographic representation of the experimental
SISI signal, as determined by a Tektronix 543A oscilloscope (Tektronix, Inc.,
Beaverton, Ore.), indicated a rise-and-fall time of 10 milliseconds and a
peak-to-peak time of 350 milliseconds, for an overall time of 357 milliseconds
($T = 2r/3 + P$; Dallos and Olsen, 1964). The 1-dB intensity increment,
predetermined by the audiometer, was found to be 1.25 dB, as indicated by a
Bruel and Kjaer sound-level meter (2203) and artificial ear (4252)[1] (Bruel
and Kjaer Instruments, Inc., Cleveland, Ohio).

The relay programming apparatus controlled the temporal interval between auditory signal presentations and the temporal characteristics of the
auditory signal. The programming apparatus also controlled the availability of
the response circuit to discriminative stimuli or control periods, as well as the
time-out periods, recorded subject responses (signal responses, control responses, and total responses), and programmed reinforcement delivery. Intertrial responses were determined by subtracting signal and control responses
from total responses. The examiner also manually recorded responses for each
trial (signal and control). The same programming apparatus can be used for
both puretone threshold and SISI measurements.

PROGRAMMING

Trials were determined by a variable-interval timer centered on a VI 6-second
schedule. Although the standard SISI procedure presents the signal on a
fixed-time schedule of 5 seconds, a variable schedule was used to control the
possibility that the subject might make temporal discriminations. The signal
(intensity increments) and control periods were delivered alternately. In
effect, SISI increments occurred on the average of one every 14 seconds if no
intertrial responses were made by the subject. The presentation program was

---

[1] To avoid short-increment stimulus ballistics with the sound level meter, the S^D
programming timer was set for 5 seconds. This permits the meter to indicate a stable
measurement for a duration sufficient to record the intensity level without ballistic
effects.

essentially the same as that used for stimulus presentation in the puretone threshold program. Responses made during the interval that the response circuit was not open (intertrial responses) delayed the occurrence (time out) of either control or signal trials. Observance of responses to control periods provided a systematic method of determining whether responses were discriminative or random. The signal and control periods maintained the same temporal characteristics. The duration of the trial periods was controlled by a timer and was preset as required for each phase of the program.

A posttone delay in the response circuit, discussed in Chapter 1, kept the response circuit open after the termination of a signal or control. The posttone delay was adjusted as required by the procedural schedule. The time-out touch plate, previously described, controlled for random intertrial responses caused by the subject's "playing" with the response button.

Responses to the signal were reinforced immediately in the same manner as for puretone thresholds.

Other than presetting of the program timers and of the intensity and frequency controls for the signal increments, the program was automatically controlled.

PROCEDURAL VALIDATION

The applicability and validity of the initially designed experimental procedure were checked by comparing it with the standard handraising, fixed-interval SISI procedure. [With a Tektronix 543 A oscilloscope, photographic analysis of the standard SISI adapter (enclosed in Allison 22) indicated a rise-and-fall time of 15 and 20 milliseconds, respectively, with peak-to-peak time of 215 milliseconds, for an overall time of 232 milliseconds ($T = 2r/d + P$; Dallos and Olsen, 1964)]. A 19-year-old, moderately retarded subject with a known bilateral, severe, sensorineural loss was used as a validation subject. The subject previously had yielded consistent, positive (100 percent) SISI scores by standard procedures.

Experimental and standard SISI procedures were presented in a counterbalanced schedule. Figure 1 illustrates a comparison of data between procedures. Results indicate that the subject detected fewer SISI signals with the experimental procedure than with the standard procedure. Occasionally, the VI 6-second interval was altered to a VI 11-second presentation to determine whether the temporal interval would affect signal detection. Results indicated no appreciable differences between the two intervals. The differences between procedures may have been due partially to the fixed standard and variable experimental intervals used in the procedures. Variable presentation schedules prevent subjects from developing temporal response patterns which

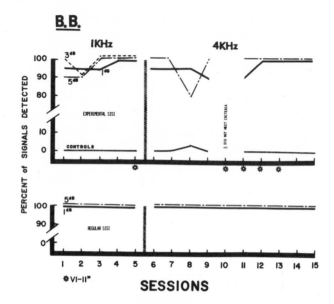

Figure 1. Responses by a mildly retarded subject to standard and experimental SISI procedures for both 1 KHz and 4 KHz. Upper, responses to experimental SISI procedures (1, 3, and 5 dB and 0-dB controls); lower, responses to standard procedures (1 and 5 dB). S, subject.

are possible under the fixed standard schedule. We concluded that the experimental procedure yielded results which were similar to those obtained with the conventional SISI test.

APPLICATION EXPERIMENT

The purpose of this experiment was to investigate the feasibility and application of an experimental procedure to a random sample of severely retarded children.

Subjects

Six severely retarded males ranging in IQ or SQ from 13 to 37 (mean, 22.5) and in chronological age 9 years, 9 months to 19 years, 6 months (mean of 16 years, 8 months) were subjects. None of the subjects was testable by standard audiometric techniques. Audiometric screening or threshold data obtained by stimulus-response control procedures had been obtained previously from all subjects. Three subjects had overall configurations of normal hearing, one a mild conductive loss, one a severe mixed loss, and one a profound sensorineural loss for the test ear.

The two subjects (with highest IQ's) with the conductive and mixed losses were unable to complete the pretraining phases (see "Pretraining Results").

Pretraining Procedures

All subjects were pretrained with an eight-phase procedure (see Table 1). Subjects were required to meet the stimulus-response control criterion for each phase. Control criterion was defined as responses to nine of 10 auditory signals with no more than one response to 10 control periods for 20 consecutive alternating trials.

Experimental SISI Program and Procedure

Individual thresholds (1 KHz) were established during the first experimental session. This became the reference threshold for subsequent program presentations at that frequency. A reference threshold was established for each

Table 1. Eight-phase SISI pretraining procedures

Phase	Signal duration (sec)	Posttone response availability (sec)	Signal intensity (dB SL)
1	3.0	0.3 (300 msec)	30
2	2.0	0.3 (300 msec)	30
3	1.0	1.0	30
4	0.5	1.5	30
5	0.357*	2.0	30
6	0.357*	1.5	30

7 Maintain signal duration program from Phase 6 and insert pedestal tone (Channel 2) at SL in test ear. Increase intensity of the pedestal tone in 2-dB steps, each time the subject meets control criterion, until the pedestal tone reaches 20 dB SL

8 Maintain pedestal tone program from Phase 7 and the signal temporal characteristics from Phase 6 and reduce the signal intensity in 2-dB steps, each time the subject meets control criterion, until the subject is 4 dB relative to pedestal tone

*Actual signal duration as determined by analyses with oscilloscope. Other durations are approximate, as determined by electromechanical timers.

frequency condition investigated immediately preceding that frequency series of sessions. Only one frequency was tested during any given experimental session. The SISI pedestal tone was delivered at 20 dB SL.

Subjects were required to meet the criterion, i.e., to respond to nine of 10 signals of 5 dB, 357 milliseconds in duration, and to no more than one of 10 controls for 20 alternating trials, in each session prior to administration of the experimental test.

The SISI increment was triggered by the electromechanical relay apparatus. Alternating signal and control trials were presented on a VI 6-second schedule. SISI increments followed a schedule of 5-3-1-1-3-5-1-1 dB (1 dB = actual 1.25 dB; the 3- and 5-dB increments were not analyzed for actual intensity because they served as control stimuli rather than as experimental discriminative stimuli) and then were recycled. A total test included 10 5-dB, 10 3-dB, and 20 1.25-dB increments, and 40 control periods.

Subjects were required to respond to the signal within 1.5 seconds (posttone delay) in order for a correct response to be recorded and reinforced. Control periods had the same temporal characteristics as the signal periods but were not reinforced.

Initially, all subjects were placed in a program using a 1-KHz signal with 5-, 3-, and 1.25-dB increments. Later, the 3-dB increments were dropped from the program and frequency was varied.

The purpose of this exploratory investigation was to examine the effects of various manipulations of independent variables and contingencies. Thus, all subjects were not examined as a function of a uniform, predetermined procedural design.

RESULTS AND DISCUSSION

Pretraining

Two subjects did not complete the pretraining phases: one subject was unable to meet the criterion for Phase 3 after nine sessions of 36 pairs of signal and control trials per session, and the second was unable to meet the criterion for Phase 8 after 37 sessions. Stimulus-response control was lost with both subjects because of what appeared to be the loss of reinforcer effectiveness.

The remaining four subjects had little difficulty in adapting to the pretraining phases. Table 2 indicates the number of signal trials required to meet the pretraining criterion. If the subject met the criterion for a particular phase early in a session, a new phase was not initiated. Instead, the training conditions (usually, 36 signal presentations) remained in effect until the end of the session. A new phase was not initiated until the following session.

Table 2. Number of signal trials required, by subject, for subjects (Experiment 1) to meet pretraining criteria for experimental SISI program

Phase	Trials to criteria/extra trials			
	R. B.	D. D.	W. G.	B. M.
1	10/26	10/–	48/–	16/20
2	10/26	10/45	10/12	10/26
3	10/26	10/–	13/23	46/26
4	10/26	10/18	34/02	28/08
5	10/26	–*/–	14/22	10/26
6	10/26	10/26	48/24	10/–
7	140/04	36/–	174/06	252/–
8	161/–	–†/–	79/–	108/–
Subtotal	361/160	86/89	420/89	480/106
Total	521	175	509	586
No. of sessions	14	6	15	16

*Program error, skipped Phase 5.

†This subject had a severe loss (100 dB); therefore, the discriminative signal was already at the prescribed level and this phase was not appropriate.

Therefore, between 15 and 30 percent of the total number of trials were not necessary to meet the criterion. It could be speculated that the extra trials enhanced quicker attainment of the criterion for the next phase; however, it is equally probable that the extra trials had little effect on the next phase. In fact, it is possible that there was an overall adverse effect.

Phases 7 and 8 required the largest number of trials. However, these phases employed several small stimulus changes, i.e., 2 dB, and required that the criterion be met for each change. Because this was the initial procedural endeavor, it seemed appropriate to change the stimulus in small increments to avoid the risk of losing stimulus-response control with the subject. Empirical observation of the pretraining data suggests that these phases probably could be modified to use 5-dB increments. That would shorten the procedure by approximately 50 percent.

This change in procedure would reduce both test time and the possibility of reinforcement satiation by the subject. Initially, subjects may be highly motivated by a reinforcer, i.e., candy, but after several sessions, it may lose its reinforcing properties. This factor, however, is variable. Control is maintained for most subjects for long periods of time, although it sometimes is lost with other subjects.

Experimental Data

Subject B. M. (see Figure 2) demonstrated poor discrimination control (detections of 3- and 5-dB increments) for the first six sessions despite the fact that he had met the stimulus-response control criterion of 5-dB increments before each test session. The subject displayed an overall "discriminative learning" effect and demonstrated a 1.25-dB detection rate within the "positive" range, i.e., 60–100 percent, by Session 9. Other than in Session 19, the subject maintained a high detection rate through Session 23. With the introduction of the 4 KHz signal, the subject's detection rate dropped to a "questionable" range, i.e., 20–65 percent, and then again demonstrated a "learning" effect. The VI schedule was changed from 6 to 11 seconds (see asterisks, Figure 2), 24 seconds between S^D's, so that stimulus presentation effects could be observed. No dramatic effects were noted. Responses to control periods did not increase as 1.25-dB detections increased. Increment detection, therefore, was not a direct function of an increase in high-rate responding.

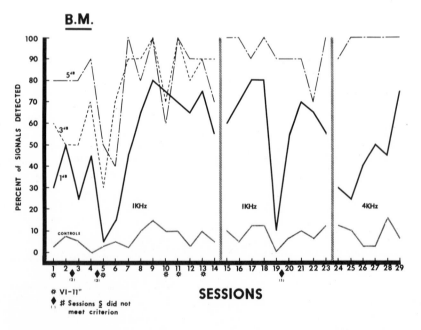

Figure 2. Responses by a severely retarded subject to experimental SISI procedures. Subject (S̲) had essentially a normal hearing configuration.

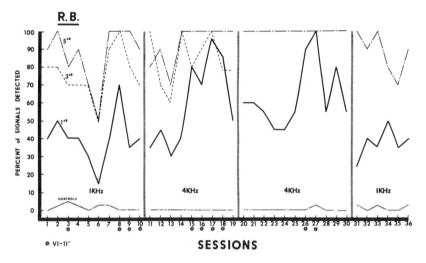

Figure 3. Responses by a severely retarded subject to experimental SISI procedures. Subject indicated normal hearing.

Subject R. B. (see Figure 3) also demonstrated variability in 3- and 5-dB increment detection during the early sessions. The increase in 1.25-dB detection scores observed with B. M. was not noted with R. B. for the 1 KHz signal but did occur with the 4 KHz signal. A return to the 1 KHz stimulus indicated a response pattern that was less variable than the initial 1 KHz presentation. The percentage of detections was similar between both 1 KHz presentations, thus suggesting that frequency was a critical variable. This finding is in agreement with published data (Harford, 1967; Yantis and Decker, 1964), indicating that SISI scores are related to signal frequency. However, the interrelated effect of signal frequency and increased scores was not expected, particularly when frequency was not a critical variable in increasing scores for B. M. (B. M. demonstrated increased scores for both 1 KHz and 4 KHz with practice). Had either of the first two subjects demonstrated sensorineural losses, it might be assumed that the detection increase was a result of inadequate pretraining, thus invalidating the initial sessions. However, because the subjects manifested normal hearing configurations and thresholds, "negative" SISI scores were expected.

Subjects D. D. and W. G. (see Figure 4), like B. M. and R. B., showed less variability in detection of the 5-dB increment as sessions progressed. However, they did not show the pronounced detection increase for the 1.25-dB increments, as had been noted with the first two subjects. Some increase in detection performance did occur, however, as evidenced by comparison of the configuration of data plots for the first and third frequency conditions

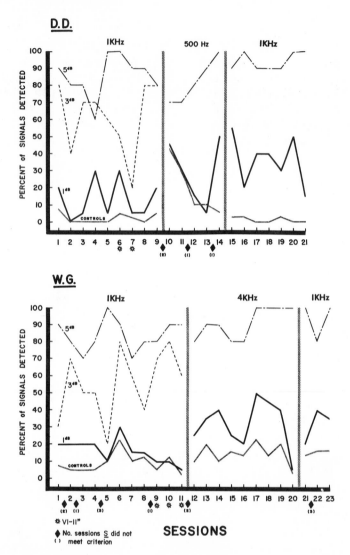

Figure 4. Responses by two severely retarded subjects (S̲) to experimental SISI procedures. D. D. had a severe sensorineural loss and W. G. had essentially normal hearing.

(both 1 KHz). Although a slight increase in increment detection was noted, the scores did not move from negative or questionable ranges to positive ranges, as had been noted with the first two subjects.

D. D.'s scores are noteworthy, inasmuch as he manifested a severe sensorineural loss, whereas the other three subjects had normal puretone thresholds (positive SISI scores are expected with cochlear sensorineural losses). However, results may have been affected by the fact that because D. D.'s threshold was 100 dB (at 1 KHz), the SISI presentation had to be made at 10 dB SL. Also, low frequencies tend to be poor indices of the SISI phenomenon. During threshold assessment, the subject did not respond to frequencies above 1 KHz at maximal limits of the audiometer, and we were forced to use 500 Hz.

The results of this experiment indicate that the experimental SISI procedure outlined is feasible with severely retarded subjects. This in itself is a significant development, in view of the complexity of stimulus contingencies imposed by the SISI task. It is also a significant observation that severely retarded individuals, heretofore relegated to gross audiologic measures, can respond to small differential stimuli, i.e., auditory signals 357 milliseconds in duration and 1.25 dB in intensity difference, on a relatively consistent and reliable basis.

The data suggest that the major issue is not one of the ability of severely retarded subjects to respond to the task but of the effects of practice on the detection of SISI signals. More specifically, the question is whether the procedure trains an increase in increment detection to a point that when subjects are under stable 5-dB stimulus control, they also are capable of 1.25 detections. If so, the question remains whether subjects with normal hearing acuity or pathologies, who theoretically should manifest negative SISI values, will improve their discriminative skills, thereby changing their diagnostic scores from negative to questionable or positive and thus indicate cochlear involvement. Jerger (1962b) hinted that improved SISI scores might result from practice effects on repeated tests; he found improvements of up to 12.3 percent (4 KHz) while measuring test-retest reliability. A subsequent experiment by Fulton and Spradlin (1972) with adults of normal intelligence supports the above findings with the retarded:

1. SISI scores increased with practice.

2. Increased SISI scores persisted after three weeks of no practice.

3. Increased SISI scores were not a function of frequency; however, the rate of increase tended to be greater for 4 KHz than for 1 KHz.

4. Increased SISI scores may be enhanced by, but are not dependent upon feedback.

Harless (1971) also found with normal hearing adults that some individuals demonstrate increased detection rates with practice, i.e., with serial tests within the same sessions.

SUMMARY

Severely retarded children can be trained to detect SISI signals. Not only are they able to respond, but they may demonstrate increased detection rates of SISI signals with practice, and, subsequently, pathologic classification may change. It is also important to note that the SISI procedures used are compatible with, and extensions of, the stimulus-response control threshold procedures. There is no reason to suspect that these same basic procedures could not be extended to difficult-to-test populations other than the retarded.

LITERATURE CITED

Dallos, P. J., and W. O. Olsen. 1964. Integration of energy at thresholds with gradual rise-fall tone pips. J. Acoust. Soc. Amer. 36: 743–751.

Fulton, R. T., and J. E. Spradlin. 1972. Effects of practice on SISI scores with normal hearing subjects. J. Speech Hear. Res. 15: 217–224.

Harford, E. R. 1967. Clinical application and significance of the SISI test. *In*: A. B. Graham (ed.), Sensorineural Hearing Processes and Disorders, pp. 223–234. Little, Brown & Co., Boston.

Harless, E. L. 1971. The effects of practice on short increment sensitivity index (SISI) scores. Unpublished master's thesis, Vanderbilt University, Nashville, Tenn.

Jerger, J. 1962a. Hearing tests in otologic diagnosis. ASHA 4: 139–145.

Jerger, J. 1962b. Comparative evaluation of some auditory measures. J. Speech Hear. Res. 5: 3–17.

Jerger, J., J. L. Shedd, and E. Harford. 1959. On the detection of extremely small changes in sound intensity. Arch. Otolaryngol. 69: 200–211.

Martin, F. N. 1972. The short increment sensitivity index (SISI). *In*: J. Katz (ed.), Handbook of Clinical Audiology, pp. 204–215. Williams & Wilkins, Baltimore.

Yantis, P. A., and R. L. Decker. 1964. On the short increment sensitivity index (SISI test). J. Speech Hear. Dis. 29: 231–246.

5 The Threshold Tone Decay Test

Robert T. Fulton and
Paul A. Waryas

Tone decay is the progressive weakening of auditory nerve fiber response as a function of time. At suprathreshold levels, perceived loudness decreases with time. At near threshold levels, perceived loudness may disappear completely. Studies concerned with the tone decay phenomenon were undertaken as early as the 19th century (Green, 1972). Interest in this phenomenon in the United States has developed only over the past 20 years. Green (1972) has written an extensive summary of the historical aspects of tone decay as well as its theoretical and clinical development. The discussion here is limited to the more recent literature in order to put the stimulus-response control procedure in perspective.

Stimulated by the work of Hallpike and Hood (1951), who distinguished between initial auditory excitation (on-effect) and progressive adaptation to continuous auditory excitation (relapse), Carhart (1957) reported a procedure developed in 1954 at Northwestern University for testing auditory adaptation at threshold. This "threshold tone decay test" has become a standard part of the basic audiometric test battery. The procedure requires the subject to raise a finger on hearing a tone and to keep it raised as long as he perceives the tone. A puretone is presented initially at 5 dB SL and subsequently is raised in 5-dB steps each time the subject lowers his finger until he perceives the tone for a full 60 seconds.

Rosenberg developed in 1958 and reported in 1969 a modification of this procedure aimed at reducing some of the test time and possible auditory fatigue involved in Carhart's method. In the Rosenberg procedure, the signal is presented for a total of 60 seconds regardless of how many 5-dB increment increases are necessary for the subject to continue to perceive the tone. The difference between the final sensation level and the original threshold was defined as the amount of tone decay present.

Green (1963) observed that instructions given to subjects influenced their results and that some subjects lost signal "tonality" before signal audibility. Therefore, he instructed his subjects to raise an arm perpendicular to an armrest if the signal was perceived as "tonal," to lower the arm 45° if tonality disappeared but audibility continued, and to lower it completely if audibility disappeared. This modification was proposed to obtain maximal sensitivity from the tone decay test.

On the basis of additional work by Hood (1950, 1955), Owens (1964) presented another modification of the tone decay test procedure. Owens' procedure was basically the same as Carhart's, except for a 20-second rest period between each 5-dB increment. It was felt that the rest period permitted the auditory system sufficient time to return to a base state. His subjects also were required to perceive the tone for a full 60 seconds at a given intensity level.

In the past 10 years, several case studies have concerned the various tone decay test modifications as they relate to each other (Parker and Decker, 1971; Sung, Goetzinger, and Knox, 1969), to other portions of the audiometric test battery, especially Bekesy audiometry (Johnson, 1965, 1970), and to specific etiologies of sensorineural dysfunction (Sorensen, 1962). When taken together, the results of these studies are somewhat confusing. No definite trend is apparent except that all of the modifications are sensitive to abnormal auditory adaptation. We are inclined to agree with the view of Katz (1969), who stated:

> Any of the three tone-decay tests [Carhart, Rosenberg, or Owens] can be used to compare performance in the better ear versus performance in the poorer ear. Specific methods employed by clinicians may vary from patient to patient and from visit to visit. Several variations may be tried with difficult cases.

The modification by Owens (1964) seems the most applicable for the development of an operant procedure for evaluating threshold tone decay of a difficult-to-test population. This modification forms the basis of the procedures we explored in our attempt to develop a tone decay test to be included in a stimulus-response control audiometric test battery. Before describing the development of the experimental tone decay test into its present form, we must reemphasize that any procedure for obtaining threshold tone decay is only one test in a battery of audiologic and medical tests necessary for proper diagnosis of retrocochlear disorders. By no means should it be the only diagnostic procedure employed.

DEVELOPMENT OF TEST MODEL

Traditional audiometric handraising procedures are usually inappropriate for difficult-to-test populations. The problem, therefore, is one of developing tone decay test procedures compatible with the existing model.

Early in the test development stages, we realized that our contention that subjects were trained by puretone stimulus-response control training procedures to respond to acoustic differences in their environments is not totally true. The subjects had been trained to respond to the "onset" of stimulus changes. We had not accounted for the "offset." We often had made provisions for those subjects who were influenced by offset but we had designed our programs around the onset. The offset response obviously is critical to the tone decay task.

After limited pilot experience with the development of the tone decay test, it was decided arbitrarily that the pretraining procedures for this task should begin with the shaping and reinforcement of offset responses. Once reasonable stimulus-response control was established to the signal offset, we then would establish stimulus-response control of the onset of the stimulus. The onset response usually was present as a result of previous training for puretone tests. If the onset response had extinguished, it rapidly returned with the reinstatement of a contingent reinforcement.

In our initial pilot investigations, we pretrained our subjects to respond consistently to the offset of an auditory stimulus. We then programmed our test stimulus (5 dB SL) to be continuously present with 200-millisecond interruptions, each 60 seconds in duration. It was postulated that if the subject with normal hearing consistently responded to the 200-millisecond interruption signal, then the ear had not adapted the 5-dB stimulus. However, if the subject did not respond, then the ear had adapted to the point at which it could not detect the offset. Initially, we were dealing only with normal-hearing subjects and we expected the responses to occur only at the 60-second interruption interval.

It was noted that, apart from the responses made in relation to the interruption each 60 seconds, there were intertrial responses. Such responses are not uncommon with this population, but they usually are brought under control with control periods and criteria. However, the usual procedures were not applicable here. We therefore proposed to bring such responses under observation by using a pen recorder to note responses and interruption events on a time base. In this way, we could determine whether an intertrial response (ITR) had a temporal base, i.e., 20 seconds after each interruption, suggesting an adaptation of 5 dB within 20 seconds. We set up a test run of 10 minutes, permitting 10 interruption events for each intensity. We assumed that consistency in response at any intertrial point would give us an adaptation pattern, particularly if the response pattern moved in relation to the intensity level of the stimulus.

Because our initial subjects indicated normal hearing, we really could not expect consistency in the temporal shifting of response patterns, resulting from adaptation, as suggested above. It was noted that the subjects responded relatively consistently to the interruption. In thinking through possible response patterns, we realized that it would be possible for subjects to adapt and respond, consistently, in less than 60 seconds and still respond to the 60-second interruption. That is, a subject could respond at the end of 40 seconds (presumably an adaptation response) yet still respond at the 60-second interval; the latter could constitute an onset response to a new stimulus, not an interruption.

It became obvious that this design was inappropriate and cumbersome and would require considerable time to administer (10 minutes per level, requiring 30–40 minutes per frequency, per ear).

We then took the task of questioning whether we could set up a design which would provide us with a wide range of information within a reasonable time. We decided on the following guidelines.

1. Subjects would be pretrained to respond within 2 seconds to both the "off" and "on" stimulus events. As previously mentioned, training would begin with off contingencies and then be combined with on contingencies once stimulus-response control had been established for off events.
2. "On" responses would serve as a control check for stimulus-response control. That is, regardless of pathology, all subjects should respond consistently to on events.
3. Arbitrary duration intervals would be instituted as checks for adaptation, i.e., off event intervals of 20, 40, and 60 seconds would be used as checkpoints for adaptation.
4. Arbitrary intensity levels would be employed as spot checks on levels of threshold adaptation, i.e., intensity levels of 15, 30, and 45 dB SL would be combined with duration intervals of 20, 40, and 60 seconds as checks of adaptation.

There is no standard classification of severity for the tone decay test (Green, 1972); however, the levels that we arbitrarily selected are reasonably related to ranges suggesting normal to mild adaptation (15 dB), mild to moderate adaptation (30 dB), and marked adaptation (45 dB).

As a result of the above guidelines, we decided on a nine-point check design or screening device to check three intervals of 20, 40, and 60 seconds at each of three intensities (15, 30, and 45 dB SL). Each point consisted of an on and off event.

We have plotted the responses that might be anticipated with varying degrees of adaptation (see Figure 1). In plotting these hypothetical functions, we have assumed that an off response is anticipated when an intensity adaptation function intersects with a line perpendicular to an interval increment. For example, the adaptation function for "B" at an intensity of 15 dB intersects only with a line that is perpendicular to the 20-second interval and not with lines that are perpendicular to the 40- or 60-second intervals; hence, off responses are anticipated only at the 20-second interval.

It should be noted that the examples presented are illustrative only. Many variations are expected. The "A" function illustrates a subject who has less than 15-dB adaptation (intersects at all nine points) and therefore would represent a person with no significant pathology. The "B" function indicates an adaptation somewhere between 30 and 45 dB and therefore has significant threshold adaptation (the only response to the 60-second increment is at the 45-dB level). The "C" function indicates a severe adaptation problem, i.e., in excess of 45 dB; even at 45 dB, the subject cannot sustain auditory perception at the 60-second interval.

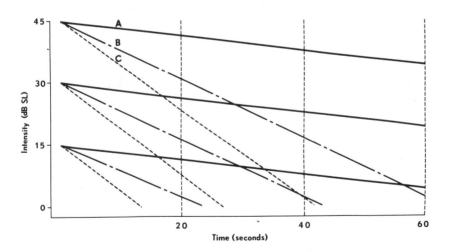

Figure 1. Hypothetical auditory adaptation functions illustrative of intensity/time interactions that might be expected from three varying degrees of adaptation (*A, B,* and *C*). When an intensity function line intersects with a line perpendicular to a time interval, a response to an offset signal could be anticipated. *A* lines (solid) indicate slight or no significant adaptation; *B* lines (broken) indicate moderate adaptation; and *C* lines (dotted) indicate severe adaptation.

To maximize the efficiency of this model, it need not be used in its entirety. For example, it would not be necessary to repeat the A function at levels above 15 dB because responses would be in evidence at all duration interval points. The model also can be extended at the discretion of the examiner. For example, the B function indicates an adaptation level of somewhere between 30 and 45 dB. The intervals could be presented at the 35- and 40-dB levels to delineate further the exact amount of adaptation. Inasmuch as the tone decay test is used for referral rather than as a tool for determining absolute values, we feel that it is more efficient to indicate a relative degree of adaptation and spend the additional time in test-retest reliability activities. The observation of on responses indicates the degree of stimulus-response control that the subject maintained during the course of the test. With the above model in mind, we set about testing its applicability.

METHOD

Subjects

Seven retarded subjects, three males and four females, were used in this investigation. The subjects ranged in age from 9 years, 7 months to 20 years, 2 months (mean of 15 years, 10 months) and in IQ from 33 to 52 (mean of 41). All subjects indicated normal hearing, as determined by operant pure-tone procedures.

Instrumentation

The same basic electromechanical programming instrumentation as that used with the puretone and SISI tests was used in this study (Appendix D). Because the test was designed to assess responses (on and off) at the nine points (three durations for each of three intensities), the durations for each intensity level were delivered in a predetermined random order. Table 1

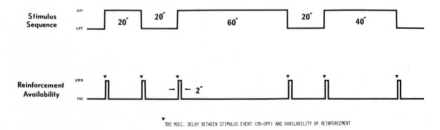

300 MSEC. DELAY BETWEEN STIMULUS EVENT (ON-OFF) AND AVAILABILITY OF REINFORCEMENT

Figure 2. Program timing sequence (in seconds) for tone decay test.

Table 1. Tape order for tone decay test
for each frequency

Intensity	Duration		
	20 sec	40 sec	60 sec
15 dB	7	8	9
30 dB	4	6	5
45 dB	2	3	1

shows the presentation order by intensity and duration for a given frequency.

Figure 2 illustrates the timing sequence. Each onset and offset event was followed by a 2-second response reinforcement period, i.e., if the subject responded to the event within 2 seconds, he was reinforced. The stimulus sequence was determined by a tape program. A 300-millisecond delay was inserted between the event and the availability of the response circuit to minimize the reinforcement of nondiscriminative responses.

Counters tabulated stimulus onset, responses to onset, stimulus offset, responses to offset, intertrial responses during stimulus on period, intertrial responses during stimulus off (silence) period, and total responses. Manual tabulation also was kept on onset and offset responses during the test period.

The stimulus frequency and intensity were generated and controlled by an Allison 22 audiometer routed through the programming apparatus. The response and reinforcement delivery apparatus was the same as that described previously for the puretone and SISI procedures. The audiometer was calibrated periodically.

Procedures

Pretraining. All pretraining was conducted at 60 dB [International Standards Organization (ISO)] with the subject's left ear. Pretraining consisted of four phases.

Phase 1. Subject responses to the offset of a 500-Hz signal were shaped with demonstrations and assistance from the experimenter as required. A manual override switch permitted the experimenter to present the signal offset at his discretion. When the subject could respond independently to the offset event, he was required to make five correct responses out of six consecutive offset presentations. This criterion was required for each of three frequencies (500 Hz, 4 KHz, and 8 KHz).

Phase 2. Responses to the onset of the signal were shaped, requiring the subject to continue to respond to the offset of the signal. Again, the experimenter presented the stimuli. To complete this phase, the subject was required to meet a 5/6 criterion (five correct responses for six consecutive presentations) for both onset and offset events for each of the three frequencies.

Phase 3. The stimulus was lengthened progressively until the subject independently could meet a 5/6 criterion for each of three randomly presented durations approximating 20, 40, and 60 seconds.

Phase 4. Training procedures then were shifted to the automatic presentation schedule, previously described, and stimuli were presented at 60 dB ISO. The subject was required to meet a 5/6 criterion for each of three frequencies.

Thresholds. Mean thresholds (500 Hz, 4 KHz, and 8 KHz; left ear) were computed from thresholds obtained during five sessions for each subject. "Threshold" was defined as the lowest level at which the subject maintained a 50-percent response rate, i.e., minimum of three correct responses, for each of six presentations.

Probe thresholds were obtained midway in the experimental sessions. If the probe threshold varied by more than ± 5 dB from the preestablished mean referent, a new mean was established.

Experimental Test Session. At the beginning of each test session, each subject was required to meet a pretest criterion to ensure stimulus-response control. To meet the criterion, subjects were required to respond correctly to five signal onsets and five offsets of six consecutive stimulus presentations. Pretest criterion presentations were presented at 45 dB SL at 500 Hz to the left ear.

Upon meeting the criterion, the subjects were presented with the experimental test, in the order presented in Figure 2, for each of three frequencies (500 Hz, 4 KHz, and 8 KHz). The order of frequency was randomized. Each subject was assessed by this procedure for six sessions.

Responses to stimulus onset and offset were recorded manually for each duration, intensity, and frequency. After each intensity level presentation, by frequency, the counters were checked, data were recorded and the counters were cleared for the next intensity level block.

Procedural Validation

The present investigators know of no report in the literature which indicates the identification of retrocochlear pathologies or auditory adaptation effects with severely retarded children. The absence of such a report should not be construed as an indication of the lack of occurrence, particularly when there has been an absence of test procedures to assist in identification.

Therefore, in an attempt to validate the procedures, a normal adult (age 51) with a known tone decay pattern was used as a validation subject. Table 2 indicates the results obtained by both the Carhart tone decay procedure and the present experimental procedure. The two procedures yielded similar results.

The responses of the subject to the experimental procedure are representative of tonality decay (Green, 1963). The subject lost tonality yet indicated that he could hear a buzzing at the end of all intervals. His responses, both motor and verbal description, suggest that serious consideration must be given Green's procedure. What is more important is what effect tonality may have on the response behavior of difficult-to-test subjects. The present investigators are currently at a loss for methods to control tonality with difficult-to-test populations.

EXPERIMENTAL RESULTS

The mean (six sessions) percentage of responses was computed for both the on and off events for each of the nine checkpoints (20-, 40-, and 60-second

Table 2. Results obtained from validation subject (normal IQ) with both Carhart (1957) and experimental tone decay procedures

Frequency	Carhart procedure (final dB SL required to sustain signal for 60 sec)	Experimental procedure (responses to nine checkpoints)			
			$20''$	$40''$	$60''$
500 Hz	5 dB	15 dB	+	+	+
		30 dB	+	+	+
		45 dB	+	+	+
		15 dB	+	−	−
4 KHz					
	10 3 trials X = 15 dB	30 dB	+	+	+
	20	45 dB	+	+	+
	15	15 dB	−	−	−
8 KHz					
	45 2 trials X = 47.5 dB				
	50	30 dB	+	−	−
		45 dB	+	+	+

durations at 15, 30, and 45 dB SL) for each of the three frequencies (500 Hz, 4 KHz, and 8 KHz) for each of the seven retarded subjects. Mean intertrial responses also were computed for both the signal (the interval during which the signal was present) and silent (the rest period interval between signals during which no signal was present) intervals for each of the intensity levels for each of the three frequencies for each of the subjects. Mean of total responses for each intensity by frequency was computed for each subject.

The range of subject means and the mean of means for all subjects (percentages) then were computed for the stimulus events (on and off events, by duration, by intensity levels, and by frequency) for the seven normal-hearing subjects (see Table 3).

No obviously significant trends were noted in the response patterns. This is as should be expected with normal-hearing nonpathologic subjects. Ideally, all normal-hearing means should indicate response patterns of 100 percent. There was a slight trend (about 50 percent of the time) for an increase of means with an increase in intensity. This was most evident at 500 Hz. This slight trend was not considered significant, particularly in view of the fact that it occurred with the on event equally as often as it did with the off event.

Seven of the 54 means (12.9 percent) indicated values below 90 percent. Six were for the off event and all seven were at an intensity level of 15 dB SL. One of these means was at 4 KHz, and the other six were divided equally between 500 Hz and 8 KHz. The overall finding was that normal-hearing retarded subjects responded to all tone decay test checkpoints better than 90 percent of the time.

As an indication of the type of stimulus-response control by the subjects, the following descriptive information on intertrial responses is presented. During the total experiment, an auditory signal was presented 1134 times for a total of 9 hours, 57 minutes, and 36 seconds. Of this time, a total of only 243 ITR's were made during the signal presentation, with an average of 40 seconds per signal. Intertrial responses by subject for each six-session experiment ranged from a total of one to 131, with a mean subject total ITR rate of 34.7 for the experiment and a median of 18. The subject with the highest response rate made over half of the total responses during signal periods. The median of subject response rates for each signal (N = 162) was .029. A total of only 56 ITR's were made during the 20-second silence periods for all subjects (N = 7) during the entire experiment (session N = 6). The mean total ITR rate during silence was eight; the median was five, ranging from 2 to 23.

Such stimulus-response control evidence is highly supportive of a statement that high performance (90 percent or better) during the on/off stimulus events was not due to nondiscriminative high-rate responding.

Table 3. Range of means and mean of means (percentage) of responses to on and off events, by stimulus duration (20, 40, and 60 sec), by intensity level of presentation (15, 30, and 45 dB SL), and by frequency (500 Hz, 4 KHz, and 8 KHz) for seven normal-hearing retarded children for six sessions each

Frequency	dB level	Stimulus duration (sec)					
		20		40		60	
		On	Off	On	Off	On	Off
500 Hz	15	67–100 (90.4)*	33–100 (80.8)	67–100 (88.0)	33–100 (90.4)	67–100 (90.4)	66–100 (88.0)
	30	83–100 (97.5)	67–100 (92.8)	83–100 (95.2)	67–100 (95.2)	67–100 (95.2)	50–100 (92.8)
	45	83–100 (97.5)	83–100 (95.1)	83–100 (97.5)	67–100 (95.2)	100–100 (100)	50–100 (92.8)
4 KHz	15	100–100 (100)	67–100 (88.0)	83–100 (97.5)	83–100 (97.5)	83–100 (97.5)	83–100 (97.5)
	30	83–100 (97.5)	83–100 (97.5)	67–100 (90.5)	83–100 (97.5)	83–100 (97.5)	83–100 (97.5)
	45	83–100 (95.1)	83–100 (95.1)	67–100 (92.8)	83–100 (95.1)	100–100 (100)	83–100 (95.1)
8 KHz	15	67–100 (92.8)	50–100 (85.5)	83–100 (92.7)	66–100 (78.4)	83–100 (92.7)	67–100 (88.0)
	30	83–100 (90.2)	83–100 (95.1)	83–100 (97.5)	83–100 (97.5)	67–100 (92.8)	100–100 (100)
	45	83–100 (95.1)	100–100 (100)	83–100 (95.1)	100–100 (100)	83–100 (97.5)	83–100 (97.5)

*Numbers in parentheses = mean of means.

Neither the application of the experimental procedure to normal hearing subjects nor its resultant data can be construed as supportive evidence of the validity of the procedure in identifying retrocochlear pathologies. However, the experiment does provide information for the process of test development and suggests deductive validity. If the rationale presented is valid, the basis of the principles of existing methodology, and the results are in agreement with known nonpathologic cases, then it might be assumed by deduction that the procedure holds promise for pathologic conditions. However, at this time, the investigators are not willing to conclude on the basis of deduction that the procedure is valid until it can be applied to known retrocochlear cases. Such hesitation should be taken not as a lack of faith but as a rule of respect for research principles. In short, the experimental procedure indicates considerable promise but needs further investigation.

At this juncture, the procedure is still rather cumbersome, particularly in relation to the pretraining procedures. To maximize interprocedure training procedures, it may be necessary to return to the initial stimulus-response control procedures for threshold training and to insert modifications, employing onset-offset response principles.

Additional investigation should be conducted on the recommended number of retests required to ensure response reliability. The procedure also should be subjected to replication and validation with pathologic populations.

Despite these qualifications, the experiment demonstrates the feasibility of tone decay procedures with difficult-to-test populations.

LITERATURE CITED

Carhart, R. 1957. Clinical determination of abnormal auditory adaptation. Arch. Otolaryngol. 65: 32–39.

Green, D. S. 1963. The modified tone decay test (MTDT) as a screening procedure for eighth nerve lesions. J. Speech Hear. Dis. 28: 31–36.

Green, D. S. 1972. Threshold tone decay. In: J. Katz (ed.), Handbook of Clinical Audiology, pp. 249–270. Williams & Wilkins, Baltimore.

Hallpike, C. S., and J. D. Hood. 1951. Some recent work on auditory adaptation and its relationship to the loudness recruitment phenomenon.

Hood, J. D. 1950. Studies in auditory fatigue and adaptation. Acta Otolaryngol. (Suppl.) 92: 1–56.

Hood, J. D. 1955. Auditory fatigue and adaptation in the differential diagnosis of end-organ disease. Ann. Otolaryngol. 64: 507–518.

Johnson, E. W. 1965. Auditory test results in 110 surgically confirmed retrocochlear lesions. J. Speech Hear. Dis. 30: 307–317.

Johnson, E. W. 1970. Auditory test results in 268 confirmed retrocochlear lesions. Internat. Audiol. 9: 15–19.

Katz, J. 1969. Differential diagnosis of auditory impairments. *In:* R. T. Fulton and L. L. Lloyd (eds.), Audiometry for the Retarded with Implications for the Difficult-to-Test, pp. 97–124. Williams & Wilkins, Baltimore.

Owens, E. 1964. Tone decay in VIIIth nerve and cochlear lesions. J. Speech Hear. Dis. 29: 14–22.

Parker, W., and R. L. Decker. 1971. Detection of abnormal auditory threshold adaptation (ATA). Arch. Otolaryngol. 94: 1–7.

Rosenberg, P. E. 1969. Tone decay. Maico Audiol. Lib. Ser. 7: 17–20.

Sorensen, H. 1962. Clinical application of continuous threshold recording. Acta Otolaryngol. 54: 403–422.

Sung, S. S., C. P. Goetzinger, and A. W. Knox. 1969. The sensitivity and reliability of three tone-decay tests. J. Audit. Res. 9: 167–177.

Applications to Psychoacoustic Research

On the basis of psychoacoustic research literature concerning normal, experienced listeners, it is obvious that the task of determining the effects of well-specified acoustic stimuli on difficult-to-test persons would not be a simple task. However, the need cannot be dismissed because of the difficulty of the task. Therefore, we initiated a program of psychoacoustic research into the response behavior of difficult-to-test persons. We began with relatively simple detection and discrimination paradigms and presented signals which varied in only one parameter, i.e., time, frequency, or intensity. Subsequent research should investigate interrelationships between parameters and binaural perception. This problem opens a whole new area of investigation into basic referents and subsequent training programs. For example, there is the question of whether it is necessary for a child to learn auditory perceptual concepts before he is capable of efficient speech and language training.

The following investigations of time, frequency, and intensity are by no means comprehensive, but they do provide some insight into a new area of research with difficult-to-test persons.

The presentation of these studies also is intended to demonstrate the further application of the stimulus-response control procedures to the study of auditory processes with difficult-to-test populations.

6 Detection of Short-Duration Signals

Robert T. Fulton and
Paul A. Waryas

Signal duration is an important variable in the perception of both speech and nonspeech auditory stimuli. Duration of consonantal phonemes can be used to distinguish plosives from fricatives (Black and Singh, 1968). Perceived stress can be influenced by vowel duration as well as by intensity (Fry, 1968). In addition, silent interval duration between phonemes may influence speech perception. Several Haskins studies (Bastian, Delattre, and Liberman, 1959; Bastian, Eimas, and Liberman, 1961; Harris, Bastian, and Liberman, 1961) have reported that the insertion of a temporal gap of approximately 50 milliseconds after the /s/ friction of the word *slit* induced the perception of /p/, that is, *split*. Liberman et al. (1961) also have shown differentiation between *rapid* and *rabid* on the basis of durational cues.

Varying effects are noted in the relation between duration and nonspeech signals. The apparent pitch of short tones decreases with decreases in duration to a pitchless click below 10 milliseconds (Ekdahl and Stevens, 1938). Loudness also decreases with a decrease in duration (Bekesy, 1938). Intensity difference limens (DL's) have been shown to increase with decreases in duration (Upton and Holway, 1938). Finally, Tobias and Schubert (1959) have reported a dependence of interaural temporal relations on stimulus duration. This last study also has implications for "competing speech" studies as well as for clinical tests of "central" auditory functioning.

Excluding cortical-evoked response audiometry, no behavioral work has been reported that used short-duration auditory stimuli with low-level retardates other than audiologic assessment with the SISI procedure (see Chapter 4). Therefore, an investigation of short-duration detection was initiated as a preliminary step in a psychoacoustic research program of basic acoustic parameters. The purpose of this series of studies was twofold: (a) to determine the response patterns of severely retarded subjects to short-duration stimuli (14–112 milliseconds), and (b) to determine whether increased detection rates ("discriminative learning") were evident across sessions, as was noted in the SISI experiments (see Chapter 4).

The investigations were divided into two parts: (a) short-duration augmentation detection, and (b) short-duration interruption detection.

SHORT-DURATION AUGMENTATION DETECTION

The purpose of this experiment was to determine the ability of severely retarded children to detect short-duration stimulus augmentations (14–112 milliseconds) of 10 dB in the presence of a continuous pedestal stimulus. The data also were analyzed for evidence of increased detection (discriminative learning) as a function of time or practice.

Method

Eight severely retarded subjects, seven males and one female, were used in this study. Subject IQ's or SQ's ranged from 25 to 40, with a mean of 32. Ages ranged from 10 to 18 years. All subjects had been tested previously with the operant puretone procedures and had indicated puretone thresholds within normal limits.

Each subject was required to meet the following pretest training criteria before the experimental program was initiated.

1. Each subject was retrained by standard puretone stimulus-response control training procedures (see Appendix A), except for phases considered non-applicable to these experiments [broad-spectrum noise generated by a Grason-Stadler audiometer (Model 162; Grason-Stadler Co., Concord, Mass.) replaced the standard narrow-band noise in Phase 5, and only a 1 KHz pedestal was used in Phase 6].

2. A procedure to train subjects to accept fixed reinforcement ratios was substituted for Phase 10 of the standard training procedure. During this phase, the reinforcement ratio was changed from CRF (continuous reinforcement) to FR-2 (reinforcement for every second correct response). Upon completion of five consecutive correct responses (5/0 criterion), the ratio was changed from FR-2 to FR-3 (reinforcement for every third correct response). The subjects then were required to meet an 18/20 criterion (18 correct responses out of 20 S^D trials) for two consecutive

days at FR-3. All eight subjects completed the above criteria and were included in the study.

All pretest training and test procedures were conducted in a sound-treated room (Industrial Acoustics Co.). Puretone signals were generated by a Hewlett-Packard audio oscillator (Model 201CR; Hewlett-Packard Co., Palo Alto, Calif.), attenuated by two Hewlett-Packard attenuators (Model 350D) and routed to the appropriate ear by a Grason-Stadler speech audiometer (Model 162). Ten-ohm button-type audioreceivers (Dyna Magnetic Devices, Model D308; Dyna Magnetic Devices, Inc., Hicksville, N. Y.) with custom standard earmolds were used instead of earphones. The frequency response of the receivers was flat between 100 Hz and 2 KHz. Receivers were used in preference to traditional earphones in order to minimize sound leakage or phone slippage if the subject moved.

Solid state circuitry [Grason-Stadler (GS)-1200 series] was used to present and control the programming and temporal aspects. This instrumentation retained the same basic functions as the previously described electromechanical instrumentation (Chapter 1) and at the same time provided greater flexibility and temporal control.

The programming and stimulus-control instrumentation is shown in Figure 1. This basic instrumentation array was used in all psychoacoustic experiments.

The programming apparatus included electronic switches to control the rise-and-fall times of the signals (10 milliseconds for the pretraining signal and 5 milliseconds for the test signal) and timers to control the duration of the short signals (between 14 and 112 milliseconds). The presentation schedule of discriminative stimuli and control periods (nonaudible periods of temporal characteristics identical to the S^D) was determined by a probability generator. Intertrial intervals were determined by a variable interval (VI) timer centered on 10-second intervals. The programmer controlled the availability of the 2-second response circuit subsequent to stimulus or control event. It also counted stimulus and control presentations and responses made during the subsequent 2-second response periods.

The response-reinforcement delivery apparatus was the same as that previously described for the audiometric procedures.

An inline frequency counter (Heathkit Model 1B-101; Heath Co., Benton Harbor, Mich.) was used to calibrate the stimulus frequency; a storage oscilloscope (Tektronix Model 564B) was used to analyze and monitor stimulus presentations and temporal characteristics. A sound-level meter (Bruel and Kjaer Type 2203) with a 2-cc coupler was used to calibrate signal

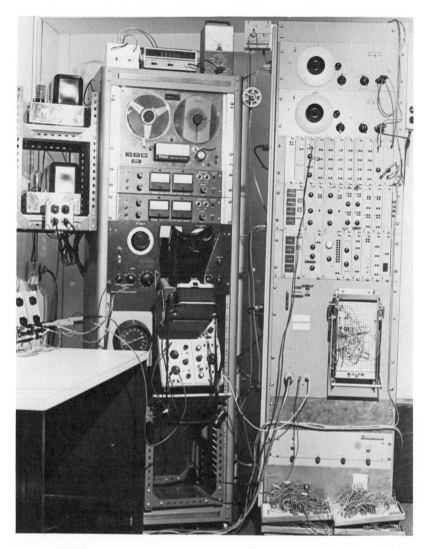

Figure 1. Instrumentation used in psychoacoustic experiments.

intensities. A block diagram of the instrumentation is shown in Figure 2, and a schematic of the GS-1200 series programming apparatus is illustrated in Appendix E.

Threshold Assessment. Mean thresholds (1 KHz; right ear) were computed from five threshold sessions for each subject. Thresholds were assessed by the descending method of Carhart and Jerger (1959). "Threshold" was defined as the lowest intensity level at which the subject maintained a 50-percent response rate, i.e., three correct responses out of six presentations. A 2-second puretone stimulus (S^D) was presented; the response circuit was "open" for 2.7 seconds (0.3 second after onset to 1.0 second after offset of the signal). The stimuli and nonaudible control events were presented randomly on a probability rate of 70/30 percent, i.e., there was a 70-percent chance that the stimulus tone would be presented and a 30-percent chance that the control period would be presented. The nonaudible control periods provided checks on random nondiscriminative responding.

Probe thresholds were reassessed after every fifth experimental test session. If the probe threshold varied by more than ± 5 dB from the preestablished mean referent, a new mean was established from three thresholds. Prior to each threshold measurement in both the initial five-session average and the probe threshold measurement, stimulus-response control was established by use of a 1 KHz, 60-dB sound pressure level 2-second signal, with a 9/10 criteria (response to nine of 10 consecutive stimulus presentations).

Pretraining. Each subject underwent a series of five pretraining phases to ensure his familiarity with the specific task and to establish his response pattern to short-duration signals of approximately 200 milliseconds.

A "continuous" pedestal tone of 1 KHz was presented at 20 dB SL. The pedestal signal served as a background from which the subjects were required to detect short-duration augmentations (S^D). The 1 KHz S^D's were presented at 30 dB SL. The pretraining schedule is given in Table 1.

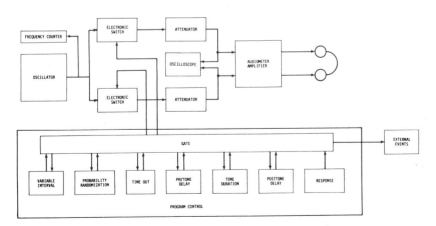

Figure 2. Block diagram of instrumentation used in the short-duration experiments.

The pretraining S^D duration (see Table 1) was decreased from 2 seconds to 200 milliseconds across five pretraining phases. The rise-and-fall time of all S^D's was 10 milliseconds. The postdelay time (additional time, following cessation of the S^D, in which a correct response could be made) was lengthened progressively as the stimulus duration was shortened. In each phase, a 90-percent minimal criterion, i.e., nine correct responses to 10 consecutive S^D presentations, was established before initiation of the succeeding phase.

Although every correct response resulted in reinforced feedback (a light in the dispenser and a door chime), edible reinforcers were delivered on a FR-3 schedule (every third correct response). The FR schedule was used to minimize subject satiation before the end of a session.

Test Sessions. Except for S^D duration and rise-and-fall times, the test stimulus parameters were essentially the same as those employed in the pretraining sessions. Subjects were required to detect short-duration 1 KHz stimuli presented at 30 dB SL in the presence of a 20-dB SL 1 KHz continuous pedestal tone.

Stimulus durations of 112, 83, 55, 31, and 14 milliseconds (with rise-and-fall times of 5 milliseconds) were used. The durations were "equivalent durations" based on the formula

$$T = \frac{2}{3}r + P$$

where T is equivalent duration, r is rise time, and P is peak time (Dallos and Olsen, 1964).

Pretest stimulus control criterion was established before initiation of each test session. The criterion required subjects to respond to a 1-KHz, 200-millisecond stimulus (10 dB relative to pedestal signal) 90 percent of the time for

Table 1. Stimulus duration pretraining presentation schedule

Phase	Approximate stimulus duration (sec)	Postdelay (sec)	Response criterion (percentage of 10 consecutive trials)
1	2.0	0.3	90
2	1.5	0.5	90
3	1.0	1.0	90
4	0.5	1.5	90
5	0.2	2.0	90

10 consecutive trials. If stimulus control was not established within 40 trials, the subject was excused for that session.

Each experimental test session consisted of five blocks of 10 presentations each, with a total of 50 trials. Each block presented a different stimulus duration (112, 83, 55, 31, and 14 milliseconds); however, the response periods were always 2.0 seconds in duration. Control periods held the same temporal relationships as did the stimulus period. Intertrial intervals, probability of presentation, and the reinforcement ratio remained the same as in the pretraining sessions.

The test blocks of 10 stimuli each were presented in one of the following orders: (a) descending order: 112, 83, 55, 31, and 14 milliseconds, (b) ascending order: 14, 31, 55, 83, and 112 milliseconds, or (c) random order by blocks. Two of the eight subjects were presented with the descending order of blocks at each session for a 10-session series, followed by the random order of blocks for a 10-session series. Two subjects were presented with the random series followed by the descending series, while two other subjects were presented with the ascending series followed by the random series. The final two subjects were presented with the random series followed by the ascending series. In the random-order sessions, the 10 stimuli within each block were identical in duration. Only the blocks were randomized. It was anticipated that the presentation schedule allowed for discussion of order of presentation effects as well as session-by-session "learning" (practice) effects.

Results and Discussion

Figure 3 presents the mean correct responses of 10 sessions and the range of correct responses for each subject as a function of duration. Stimulus durations appear across the abscissa and mean correct response appears across the ordinate; mean correct response multiplied by 10 indicates the percentage of correct responses. Each curve identifies subject and block order of presentation, with two subjects for each order.

A primary finding of this study was that low-level mentally retarded subjects detected more than 50 percent of the short-duration signals (as short as 14 milliseconds). In fact, the data in Figure 3 indicate only 11 data points below the 50-percent level (five correct responses). These 11 points constitute 13.7 percent of the total 80 data points. The majority (seven) of these low means were obtained from one subject T. K.

A second finding was that differential detection was a function of duration. Inspection of the mean curves for all of the subjects indicates that, as stimulus duration decreased, detection also tended to decrease. This was particularly evident in view of the pretest 200-millisecond response data,

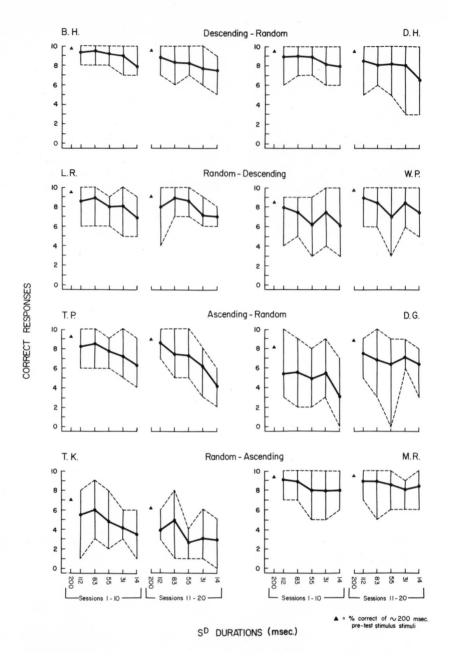

Figure 3. Mean and range of individual subject signal detections by signal duration and order of presentation (two subjects per order). Closed triangles represent the percentage (8   80%) of identifications made by each subject during the pretest identification criterion phase. Each mean indicates the mean number of detections of that duration for 10 sessions per order of presentation.

obtained from pretest criterion data. The percentages of correct detections of the total number of 200-millisecond stimuli presented were transformed

$$\left(\frac{\text{percentage of correct total 200-millisecond events}}{10} \right)$$

to fit the 0–10 scale used for the main body of the data and are represented by the closed triangles in Figure 3. The percentages of correct responses to the 200-millisecond stimuli were consistently higher than the mean detection data for all test durations.

Table 2 shows the mean detections averaged over all subjects and orders of stimulus presentation, namely, random, descending, and ascending. Because all subjects were given a series of random-order blocks as well as a directional order, the random-order category presents data for all eight subjects, whereas the ascending- and descending-order categories present the data for four subjects each. The random and descending data show a decrease in detection as a function of decreasing stimulus duration. The trend, however, is less evident for the ascending order.

The descending order of presentation produced better detection performance than the random order, which in turn produced better performance than the ascending order. However, because of the small subject sample, care must be taken in making such a generalized statement. The random-order category was composed of eight subjects, whereas the ascending- and descending-order categories were composed of four subjects each.

Figure 4 shows the range and means (pooled durations) of correct responses for the 20 test sessions. Learning effect patterns as a result of practice were anticipated; however, no trend was evident for the 20 sessions. The detection performance of two subjects (W. P. and D. G.) improved

Table 2. Mean of mean subject responses (for 10 stimulus events) by stimulus duration and order of presentation

Order of presentation	Stimulus durations (msec)				
	112	83	55	31	14
Descending (4)*	8.6	8.1	8.0	7.8	6.8
Random (8)	7.9	7.6	6.9	6.8	6.0
Ascending (4)	6.6	6.9	6.0	6.0	5.2

*Numbers in parentheses = number of subjects.

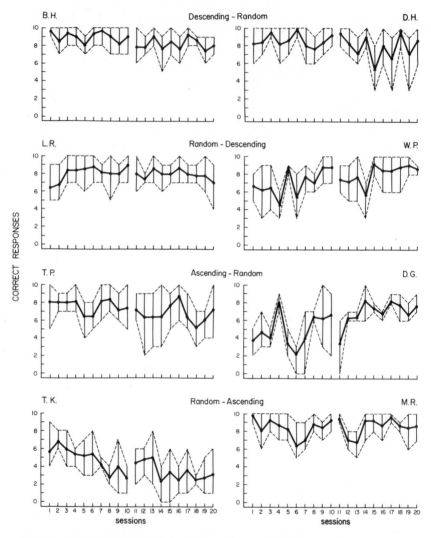

Figure 4. Range and mean of correct responses for all duration conditions by session, subject and condition presentation order.

slightly, while the performance of one subject (T. K.) deteriorated. The remaining subjects showed no change across sessions. It appeared that the high variability of responses of individual subjects, both intrasession and intersession, eliminated any possibility of demonstrating learning or practice effects.

We reasoned that the insertion of more easily perceptible stimulus durations (200 milliseconds) within each block would assist the subject in maintaining attention throughout the task and assist the experimenter in checking for stimulus-response control within the session. For this reason, two subjects (D. G. and T. K.) with the most variable range of performance were administered a modified 10-session program of duration detection.

Stimulus and reinforcement parameters of the modified program remained the same as those in the original study. The modified design differed from the original design in that two 200-millisecond stimuli were inserted randomly within each block of 10 duration signals, with a total of 12 signals per block. The five stimulus duration blocks were presented randomly for each of the 10 sessions. The 200-millisecond stimuli were used as response control checks within test sessions, in addition to the demonstrated pretest criterion performance of detecting the 200-millisecond signal preceding each test session.

The random presentation of the two 200-millisecond stimuli within each of the five duration blocks provided a vehicle to see whether stimulus control was maintained, as well as a vehicle for the total or partial acceptance or rejection of data on the basis of subject stimulus-response control. If more than 20 percent (two out of 10) of the total 200-millisecond stimuli were missed, stimulus control was considered lost and the data for the entire session were rejected. If, in any given block, both 200-millisecond stimuli controls were missed, that block was repeated at the end of the session. If, on any two given blocks, both the 200-millisecond stimulus controls were missed, the session was terminated. If the data of a given session were rejected or if the session was terminated early, the presentation schedule was repeated during the next session.

The modified program resulted in totally different behaviors by the two subjects. One subject (D. G.) completed the design in 10 consecutive sessions without the repetition of a single block within a session. A comparison of D. G.'s performance between the initial experiment and the "extension" experiment indicated improved performance (approximately 20 percent better) with decreased variability. Durations and mean responses were as follows: 112 milliseconds, 9.9; 83 milliseconds, 9.8; 55 milliseconds, 9.9; 31 milliseconds, 9.1; and 14 milliseconds, 9.1. The greatest range of variability was 7–10 for the 14-millisecond duration.

The second subject (T. K.) completed only eight of 23 sessions. Session one was presented five times before the data were acceptable; session two was presented once; session three, twice; session four, eight times; session five, three times; session six, twice; and sessions seven and eight, one time each. A comparison of T. K.'s responses between the two experiments indicated some improvement (approximately 20 percent) in mean detections; however, no appreciable improvement was made in the range of responses. Mean responses for the eight-session extension ranged from 7.25 (83 milliseconds) to 4.87 (31 milliseconds).

The subject (D. G.) who improved in performance did so in a short time. The performance of T. K. was poor and indicated little difference from that of the original study. Additional research should be conducted to assess the value of using a modified intrasession control (probe) procedure, in terms of both subject stimulus-response control and total test time involved.

In summary, the results of the short-duration augmentation detection experiments indicated that:

1. Low-level mentally retarded children could be conditioned to detect short-duration signals.
2. Detection performance tended to decrease with a decrease in signal duration.
3. Practice effects were not evident in relation to repeated testing.
4. There is a possibility that the random inclusion of two stimulus-response control presentations of 200 milliseconds within each duration block would improve subject performance.

It should be noted, however, that the durational variables investigated are subject to intensity influences. The discriminative stimulus was presented 10 dB in relation to a reference pedestal stimulus.

SHORT-DURATION INTERRUPTION DETECTION

It has been shown that the insertion of silent intervals in words results in perceptual word differences. Therefore, it was the purpose of this study to investigate the response patterns of the same subjects in detecting silent intervals, i.e., interruptions, of a continuous signal. The experimental results also are compared with pilot data obtained from normal adults, using the same durations.

Method

The same eight severely retarded subjects who were employed in the augmentation detection study also were used in this study.

The instrumentation in this study was the same as that used in the preceding study. Switch positions (see Appendix C, Plate 3) were changed to accommodate the interruption in place of the augmentation.

Threshold Assessment. Mean thresholds were computed from five thresholds (1 KHz; right ear) for each subject. The specific procedures remained identical to those in the preceding study.

Pretraining. Since the subjects moved directly from the augmentation study to the interruption study, the total pretest training program was not repeated. The number of pretraining sessions was reduced from five to three because the subjects were considered to be highly trained. The subjects began their pretraining with Phase 3, as described in the previous study, except that the continuous pedestal was presented at 30 dB SL and the subjects were required to identify each stimulus interruption (S^D).

Test Stimuli. Subjects were required to detect short interruptions (14, 31, 55, 83, and 112 milliseconds) in a 30-dB SL 1-KHz continuous pedestal tone. The fall time of the pedestal to the interruption and the rise time from the interruption to the pedestal was 5 milliseconds.

Each subject was presented with stimulus block orders identical to those that they received in the previous study.

Results and Discussion

This study indicates a direct relationship between detection and duration, similar to the previous study; however, there was a lower detection performance. The means and range of correct identifications as a function of duration are presented in Figure 5, which is the interruption duration corollary of Figure 3.

This study demonstrated a significant differential detection as a function of duration. With few exceptions, the mean number of detected interruptions decreased with the decrease in stimulus durations. The 200-millisecond stimulus pretraining data were consistently higher than any mean experimental test data point. The trend of decreased detection with the decrease in duration was least evident for two subjects. One subject (T. K.) consistently detected the fewest stimuli. This subject also gave the poorest response in the augmentation detection experiment. The other subject (M. R.) consistently detected the greatest number of stimuli. It is interesting to note that both of these subjects were given the same stimulus order (random-ascending).

As a general rule, the 55-millisecond interruption was detectable more than 50 percent of the time. This finding may be significant in view of the perceptual effects, noted by the Haskins studies, with 50-millisecond interruptions, as discussed in the introduction to this chapter.

Comparison of the mean responses in Figure 5 with those of Figure 3 indicates poorer performance in detecting short interruptions than short augmentations. The trend of decreased performance with decreased stimulus durations was much stronger in the interruption-detection study than in the augmentation-detection study.

The detection performance of the test group in the interruption study also was analyzed in terms of total mean of correct responses (average of all

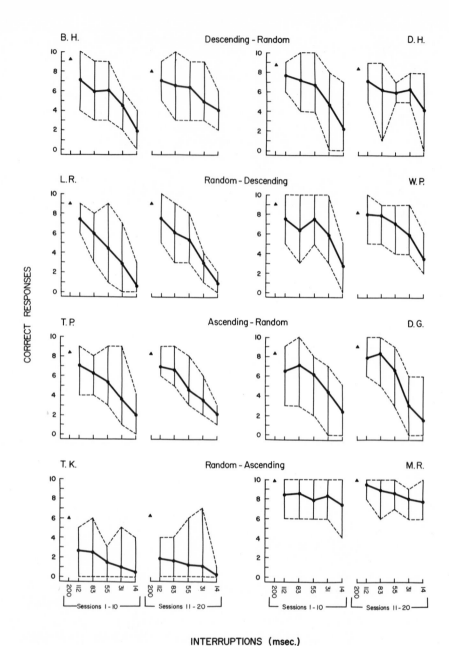

INTERRUPTIONS (msec.)

Figure 5. Mean and range of individual subject interruption detections by duration of interruption and order of presentation (two subjects per order). Closed triangles represent the percentage (8 = 80%) of detections made by each subject during pretest criterion phase. Each mean indicates the mean number of detections of each duration condition for 10 sessions per order of presentation.

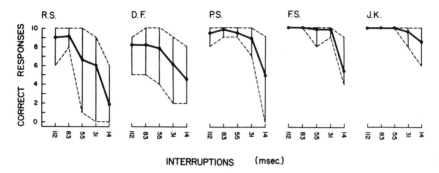

Figure 6. Mean and range of interruption detections (normal adult subjects) by duration of interruption. Data represent eight sessions of random-block presentations.

durations) and range of correct responses across the 20 sessions. The data are not presented because they are very similar to those in Figure 4. No learning or practice trend developed over the 20 sessions, and, as indicated in Figure 5, mean correct responses were generally lower in the interruption-detection study than in the augmentation-detection study.

The experimental interruption data also can be compared with pilot data obtained with five normal-hearing adult subjects of normal intelligence. The pilot data, given in Figure 6, give means and ranges of responses for eight sessions of random-block-order stimulus presentations. The pilot data also show essentially decreasing performance with a decrease in stimulus duration. More important, however, is that the response curves for two of the normal adult subjects (R. S. and D. F.) are nearly identical to the response curves for two of the retarded subjects (D. G. and W. P., respectively). Also, the best responder in the experimental test group of retarded subjects (M. R.) had a higher mean correct resonse for the shortest interruption (14 milliseconds) than all but one of the pilot subjects (normal adults).

A comparison of experimental test data and pilot data indicates (a) similar mean response trends by duration, (b) nearly identical curves obtained from two retarded and two normal adult subjects, and (c) higher mean performance by one retarded subject than by all but one of the normal subjects for the shortest interruption.

It appears that some retarded subjects can detect short-duration interruptions as well as normal subjects.

In summary, the interruption experiment indicates that:

1. Detection performance is related directly to stimulus duration, i.e., detection performance decreases as duration decreases. This relationship also held for the normal subjects in the pilot study.

2. Detection performance is lower for detecting short interruptions than for short augmentations.
3. Some low-level mentally retarded children detect short interruptions as well as normal adults.

LITERATURE CITED

Bastian, J., P. C. Delattre, and A. M. Liberman. 1959. Silent interval as a cue for the distinction between stops and semivowels in medial position [Abstr.]. J. Acoust. Soc. Amer. 31: 1568.

Bastian, J., P. D. Eimas, and A. M. Liberman. 1961. Identification and discrimination of a phonemic contrast induced by silent interval [Abstr.]. J. Acoust. Soc. Amer. 33: 842.

Bekesy, G. V. 1938. Uber die horsamkeit der ein- und ausschwingvorgange mit berucksichtigung der raumakustik. In: S. S. Stevens and H. Davis (eds.), Hearing: Its Psychology and Physiology. John Wiley & Sons, New York.

Black, J. W., and S. Singh. 1968. The psychological basis of phonetics. In: B. Malmberg (ed.), Manual of Phonetics. North-Holland Publishing, Amsterdam.

Carhart, R., and J. Jerger. 1959. Preferred method for clinical determination of pure-tone thresholds. J. Speech Hear. Dis. 24: 330–345.

Dallos, P. J., and W. O. Olsen. 1964. Integration of energy at threshold with gradual rise-fall tone pips. J. Acoust. Soc. Amer. 36: 743-751.

Ekdahl, A. G., and S. S. Stevens. 1938. The relation of pitch to the duration of a tone. In: S. S. Stevens and H. Davis (eds.), Hearing: Its Psychology and Physiology. John Wiley & Sons, New York.

Fry, D. B. 1968. Prosodic phenomena. In: B. Malmberg (ed.), Manual of Phonetics, pp. 365–410. North-Holland Publishing, Amsterdam.

Harris, K. S., J. Bastian, and A. M. Liberman. 1961. Mimicry and the perception of a phonemic contrast induced by silent interval: Electromyographic and acoustic measures [Abstr.]. J. Acoust. Soc. Amer. 33: 842.

Liberman, A. M., K. S. Harris, P. D. Eimas, L. Lisker, and J. Bastian. 1961. An effect of learning on speech perception: The discrimination of durations of silence with and without phonemic significance. Lang. Speech 4: 175–195.

Tobias, J. V., and E. D. Schubert. 1959. Effective onset duration of auditory stimuli. J. Acoust. Soc. Amer. 31: 1595–1605.

Upton, M., and A. H. Holway. 1938. On the psychophysics of hearing. I. Monaural differential sensitivity and exposure time. In: S. S. Stevens and H. Davis (eds.), Hearing: Its Psychology and Physiology. John Wiley & Sons, New York.

7 Detection of Frequency Differentials

Robert T. Fulton and
Paul A. Waryas

The frequency difference limen (DL), i.e., minimal detectable frequency change, has been studied extensively since the beginning of the 19th century. As Harris (1969) reports, "by 1900 a most impressive body of relevant papers was extant . . . from Delezenne in 1826 to Seashore in 1899." Priot to 1931 (Shower and Biddulph), however, no investigator was able to measure DL's adequately at all audible frequencies and at all intensity levels. Two major findings were reported by Shower and Biddulph: (a) relative DL's were found to be constant at frequencies above 500 Hz, and (b) absolute DL's were found to be approximately constant below 500 Hz.

PROCEDURAL VARIABLES

Although the Shower and Biddulph data have been proven reliable by replication studies since 1931, their validity has been questioned seriously (Harris, 1948, 1952) because of the procedures employed. The pitch-modulation technique used by Shower and Biddulph smoothly varied the frequency between the standard and the variable stimuli. This technique could have resulted in stimulus artifacts not present in Harris' pitch-memory technique, a method of constant stimulus differences in which subjects were required to indicate whether the second stimulus in a stimulus pair was higher or lower than the first. The data from Harris' method of constant stimulus differences show frequency DL's less than half as large as those obtained with the ABX psychophysical method, in which subjects indicate whether the third stimulus in a set is more like the first or the second stimulus (Rosenblith and Stevens, 1953).

In addition to the problems of validity with psychophysical methods, procedural variables within such a method can influence results. Daniloff et al. (1964) have shown that the Δf increment size and number of Δf variables from the referent stimulus can influence the size of the resultant DL. Subject populations also affect DL size (Harris, 1952; Riach, 1967). These findings have led us to use a modified method of constant stimulus differences with two populations, a normal-intelligence adult population and a severely mentally retarded child population. We felt that even if the results obtained from the normal subjects differed from those reported in the literature, we would be able to compare them with the results obtained from retarded subjects, since comparable procedures would be used.

RELATIONSHIP TO SPEECH AND LANGUAGE

Lieberman (1967) has hypothesized that speech perception involves categorical decisions influenced by the phonemic distinctions of the language. This implies that gross differential judgments of acoustic speech stimuli are influenced by linguistic factors. Flanagan (1957), however, has hypothesized that speech perception is based on absolute judgments of the acoustic signal. This also implies gross differential judgments, but not those involving extra-acoustic factors. Whether speech perception involves categorical decisions influenced by linguistic parameters or absolute judgments based solely on the nature of the acoustic signal, the ability to make differential judgments is basic to the process of speech perception.

Several investigators (Flanagan, 1957; Flanagan and Saslow, 1958; Henning, 1966; Michaels, 1957) have used complex acoustic signals to obtain magnitudes of discriminatory capacity comparable with those used in speech perception. Complex signals used in traditional differential threshold paradigms have yielded discriminations finer than those hypothesized by Lieberman or Flanagan but less discrete than those obtained from simple puretone DL studies.

It is possible that before determining the discriminatory capacity of a retarded population with respect to complex or speech signals, we should employ simple puretone signals to determine the maximal discriminative ability of the auditory system of these subjects. It is important to determine discriminative ability of specific parameters of the acoustic signal because we do not know the relationship between these parameters in the complex speech signal. We also do not know what acoustic information is ignored in judgments of these complex signals. Furthermore, to a large extent, we are dealing with a retarded population which, because of the lack of development of a linguistic system, may not have the ability to make linguistic categorical perceptual judgments. In order to compare the auditory functioning of retardates with that of normals, therefore, it is necessary to use stimuli which do not permit linguistic factors to influence judgments by either population.

SUMMARY

In summary, the differential threshold for frequency is an inverse measure of discriminatory capacity, i.e., the smaller the DL, the greater the discriminatory capacity. Comparable discrimination by a retarded and a normal population to a frequency DL task would suggest comparable discriminatory capacity. Moreover, comparable frequency DL performance by a retarded and a normal population would indicate that the retarded population is capable of making discriminations that are finer than necessary for speech perception.

The specific purposes of this study were twofold: (a) to compare the results of a modified method of constant stimulus difference with results of more traditional methods reported in previous studies, and (b) to compare the results obtained with normal and severely retarded subjects.

METHOD

Subjects

Two groups of subjects were used in this study, a normal intelligence group and a severely retarded group. The five normal subjects were adult female staff members who ranged in age from 21 years, 7 months to 24 years, 3 months. Puretone thresholds obtained from each at 1 KHz (right ear) were within normal limits. Only four of the five retarded subjects initially selected for this study were used. The fifth subject was unable to complete the pretraining phases after 5 weeks of training and was dropped from the study. The four remaining retarded subjects, all of whom were male, ranged in age from 14 years, 1 month to 18 years, 10 months, and in IQ's from 29 to 40. Their 1-KHz puretone thresholds (right ear) were within normal limits.

Instrumentation

All pretraining and experimental test procedures were conducted in a sound-treated room (Industrial Acoustics Co.). The apparatus used in this experiment was basically the same as that employed in the duration-detection investigation reported in Chapter 6.

The stimuli were calibrated at the acoustic output, i.e., the receiver, with a sound-level meter (Bruel and Kjaer Type 2203) and 2-cc coupler, and were analyzed and monitored with an oscilloscope (Tektronix Model 564 B), a frequency counter (Heathkit Model 1B-101), and a volt meter (Heathkit Model AV-3). A block diagram of the instrumentation used is shown in Figure 1, and a schematic diagram of the programming used appears in Appendix F.

The retarded subjects received stimuli by 10-ohm button receivers (Dyna Magnetic Devices Model D308) and custom standard earmolds. The normal subjects received all stimuli by standard TDH-39 earphones with MX 41/AR cushions. Stimuli were presented only to the right ears of the subjects. Left ears were covered with either dummy receivers and earmolds or earphones, depending on the subject group.

Procedure

Psychophysical Method. The reference signal (1 KHz) consisted of 200-millisecond pulses, with 10-millisecond rise-and-fall times and 50-percent duty cycles (200 milliseconds "on" and 200 milliseconds "off"). The reference signal was presented at 30 dB SL.

The discriminative stimuli varied from the referent stimulus only in the frequency domain. Pulse duration, duty cycle, rise and fall time, and sensation level settings were identical to those used for the standard stimulus.

The retarded subjects were presented with a larger range of frequency-increment stimuli than were the normals. The retarded also received seven-pulse discriminative stimuli, whereas normal subjects received five-pulse discriminative stimuli. This was done because pilot work indicated that the average response latency of the retarded population was slightly over 2

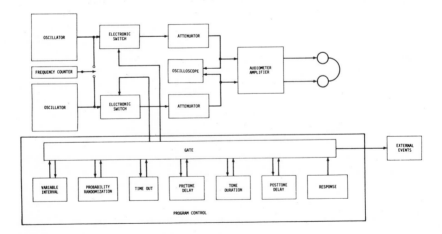

Figure 1. Block diagram of frequency DL instrumentation.

seconds (five pulses) and because the available instrumentation could not be programmed to provide a postdelay response period, as had been done in other previous experiments. Figure 2 depicts the timing sequences used for the two populations.

The combination of the referent and discriminative stimuli represented a modified method of constant stimulus differences. Instead of a subject's having to decide whether the second stimulus in a pair is higher or lower than the first, he is required only to detect the presence of a frequency difference of what amounts to the second stimulus in a pair.

Training Procedures and Reinforcement. We originally planned to pre-train the normal and retarded subjects in exactly the same manner. No verbal instructions were to be given. The pretraining procedures were to be divided into six phases. Phase 1 would consist of handshaping subject responses to 1050-Hz stimuli presented on a VI-10 schedule. Subjects then were required to meet a criterion of 90 percent correct response to 10 events by themselves before moving to the second phase. Phases 2–5 were to be identical to Phase 1 in procedure, except that the stimuli used 1025-, 975-, 1010-, and 990-Hz signals, respectively. Phase 6 consisted of four sessions of practice with the actual test stimuli to maximize subject response stability before the experimental test sessions were initiated. Correct responses were reinforced on a FR-3 schedule with nickels for the normal subjects and with subject-selected edibles for the retarded subjects.

After quickly meeting criteria in each of the five pretraining phases described above, the normal subjects exhibited varied and inconsistent response strategies during Phase 6. Some subjects responded many times during a given session, resulting in a high number of intertrial responses (ITR's). Other subjects seldom responded, resulting in larger DL's (70-percent detection points) than expected. Still other subjects shifted their response rates both within and between sessions. It was felt that subject variability was a consequence of lack of experience with the task and inadequate control of the reinforcement contingencies.

A set of written instructions was introduced to ensure a high level of attention throughout the listening sessions and to eliminate constantly changing response strategies.

The instructions for the normal subjects were as follows:

We have a pretest phase that prepares you for listening. You must meet a high correct response criteria before you can be given the test; therefore, it is to your advantage to listen hard so you meet the criteria and move to the actual test. You will not be paid for correct responses during this phase.

There are five test blocks of varying degrees of acoustic difficulty. Each block consists of a number of actual acoustic differences and a

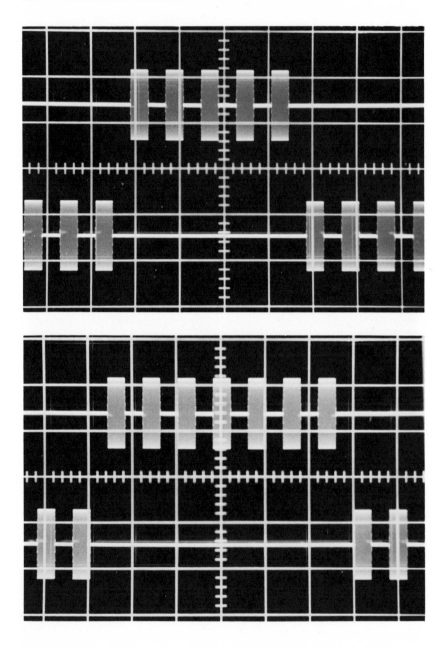

Figure 2. Timing sequences. The sequence illustrated on the top was used with the retarded subjects and the sequence on the bottom was used with the normal subjects.

number of acoustic nondifferences with intertrial intervals between events. Intertrial intervals and acoustic nondifference events are perceptually the same.

You will be paid 5¢ for each correct response to an actual acoustic difference, but if you fail to respond correctly at least once in each block, you will be fined 5¢. Each time the reinforcement apparatus lights up, it represents a correct response.

If you respond to more than one acoustic nondifference, you will be fined 5¢ for each time thereafter. There is no feedback for responses to acoustic nondifferences.

Each block will be tabulated independently by the examiner and total value will be given at the end of the session. You will not be told how you do on each block.

It can be seen from these instructions that several contingencies were changed from the original training and reinforcement plan: (a) the pretest criterion phase was not reinforced, (b) the reinforcement ratio was changed from a FR-3 to a FR-1 schedule (every correct response reinforced), (c) penalties were imposed for high rates of nondiscriminative responding as well as for not responding, and (d) although each correct response was reinforced by a light and bell from the reinforcement delivery apparatus, no money was delivered until the end of each session.

This procedure was adopted because there was no provision with our present equipment to overtly program negative reinforcement contingencies into the proposed design, i.e., to subtract a reinforcement unit from the accumulated units.

Because the subjects had performed well during the initial five pretraining phases, they were not repeated. Pretraining Phase 6 (practice) was identical to the first four test sessions; thus, it enabled us to determine after four sessions whether the response rates of the subjects had stabilized. The response rates did stabilize during this phase and the experimental test sessions were presented.

The retarded subjects posed an entirely different problem; they were experienced with the basic response procedure and naive to the development of independent strategies. The normal subjects initially attempted to develop their own varying strategies for achieving maximal reinforcement. This attempt resulted in shifting and variable response rates.

The retarded tended to respond late to the five-pulse stimuli and to demonstrate a high degree of variability in the correct number of responses for a given stimulus frequency. Also, none of the retarded subjects was able meet the criterion, as originally designed, for all of the pretraining sessions. The problem of late responses by the retarded to the five-pulse stimuli was solved by increasing the number of stimulus pulses from five to seven. In this study, the response circuit availability, i.e., the time when the subject could be reinforced for responding, was not a separate entity from the stimulus presentation timing circuit, as had been the case in other studies. The five-pulse, 2-second response period was not long enough for most of the retarded subjects. The seven-pulse stimulus lengthened the response period time to 2.8 seconds and, in turn, alleviated the late response problem.

The problems of response variability and inability to meet criteria with the retarded were more difficult to solve. The frequency difference between the discriminative stimulus and the reference signal was increased to a point at which the subjects could meet a 90-percent response criterion; then was decreased in small steps. This process required between 18 and 44 sessions (two per day) for the four retarded subjects used in the study. By the end of the pretraining sessions, all four subjects consistently responded (90-percent correct response to 10 consecutive trials) to a differential stimulus 15 Hz above and 15 Hz below the reference frequency of 1 KHz. The fifth subject did not meet the criteria after 50 test sessions and was dropped from the study.

The program contingencies for the retarded subjects differed from those of the normal subjects. The retarded subjects continued to use a FR-3 reinforcement ratio. However, because of the reinforcement and instrumentation constraints imposed, a negative reinforcement consequence could not be used with high-rate intertrial responses or high-rate control responses. If and when these high rates occurred during the pretraining sessions, corrective manual procedures, i.e., interruption of stimulus presentation (time-out) until the high-rate responses were extinguished, were employed.

The two populations did differ in procedure as a function of contingency application.

Stimulus Presentation. The experimental test sessions were divided into two conditions. Condition A consisted of stimuli at frequencies above or equal to the referent stimulus frequency of 1 KHz. Condition B consisted of stimuli at frequencies below or equal to the referent stimulus frequency. Subjects were scheduled twice daily. Group assignments of subjects were alternated and counterbalanced, i.e., subjects were presented with Condition A stimuli in the morning and with Condition B stimuli in the afternoon on odd days; this pattern was reversed on even days.

Subjects were required to meet a 90-percent (of 10 consecutive discriminative stimulus trials) criterion prior to initiation of each experimental test session in order to establish stimulus-response control. The criterion stimuli for the normal subjects were 1010 Hz for Condition A and 990 Hz for Condition B, whereas the stimuli for the retarded subjects were 1015 and 985 Hz, respectively. Control periods of acoustic nondifferences from the refence signal and of the same temporal characteristics as the discriminative stimuli were inserted as control checks of discriminative response. The discriminative stimuli, as well as control pulses, were presented on a VI 10-second schedule. The discriminative stimulus events and the control events were programmed on a 70–30 percent probability of occurrence, respectively.

The experimental test was composed of blocks of 10 stimulus events per block. The test blocks were presented in random order for 10 sessions for each condition (A or B). The normal subjects received five stimulus blocks at 1008, 1006, 1004, 1002 Hz, and 1 KHz for Condition A and five blocks at 992, 994, 996, 998 Hz, and 1 KHz for Condition B. The retarded subjects received seven stimulus blocks for each condition, i.e., the same five, per condition, received by the normal subjects plus 1012 and 1010 Hz for Condition A and 988 and 990 Hz for Condition B.

RESULTS AND DISCUSSION

A major purpose of this study was to compare the results obtained by a modified method of constant stimulus differences with results obtained by more traditional psychophysical methods. This comparison appears in Table 1.

As seen in this table, the mean frequency DL's obtained from the normal subjects are comparable with the data obtained by Shower and Biddulph (1931). The normal subject mean DL is close to the median DL that Harris (1952) obtained with untrained subjects. The mean and median DL's for the retarded subjects are close to but slightly smaller than those obtained by Riach (1967) with high-school students.

Table 1 indicates that the modified method of constant stimulus differences used in this study produces frequency DL's which are in general agreement with previous studies. In fact, variability is greater as a result of subject populations than as a result of the psychophysical method employed.

The differences in frequency DL's obtained with the two populations in this study can be observed most easily in Figure 3. The percentage of correct judgments as a function of the frequency difference between the referent (1-KHz) stimulus and the discriminative stimuli is plotted.

Each data point around the solid curve represents the mean percentage of correct judgments (100 stimuli over 10 sessions) of the five normal subjects. The closed circles represent stimulus frequencies for Condition A (1 KHz, 1002, 1004, 1006, and 1008 Hz). The closed squares represent stimulus frequencies for Condition B (1 KHz, 998, 996, 994, and 992 Hz).

Each data point around the broken-line curve represents the mean percentage of correct judgments (100 stimuli over 10 sessions) for the four retarded subjects. The open circles represent stimulus frequencies for Condi-

Table 1. Comparison of frequency DL data obtained with 1-KHz reference stimuli

Author	Method	dB SL	Statistic	N	DL
Shower and Biddulph (1931)	Limits	40	Mean	10	3.6
Harris (1952)	Constant stimulus differences	30	Individual	3 Well-trained	1.00 1.30 1.65
		30	Median	60 Untrained	3.61
Rosenblith and Stevens (1953)	Constant stimulus differences	30	Individual	2 Well-trained	1.2 3.5
	ABX	30	Individual	2 Well-trained	2.5 8.9
Riach (1967)	2 Alternative forced choice	40	Median	400 High-school	8.2
		40	Median	20 University	4.7
Fulton and Waryas	Modified constant stimulus differences	30	Mean* Median†	5 Normal 5 Normal	3.35 3.55
			Mean* Median†	4 Retarded 4 Retarded	7.90 7.15

*Mean of combined means (above and below reference stimulus).
†Median of combined DL's (above and below reference stimulus).

tion A (1 KHz, 1002, 1004, 1006, 1008, 1010, and 1012 Hz), and the closed triangles represent stimulus frequencies for Condition B (1 KHz, 998, 996, 994, 992, 990, and 988 Hz).

The curves were fitted visually to the data. The point of intersection between the curves and the 70-percent correct judgment line is close to the computed mean DL's for both populations (see Table 2.)

One interesting observation can be made in comparing the two curves. The normal (solid) curve follows the path of the traditional psychophysical function, resembling a cumulative normal distribution of values. The retarded (broken line) curve more closely approximates a linearly increasing straight-line function. The difference between these two curves suggests that the retarded may have less well-defined perceptual capabilities than the normal population even though the retarded DL's closely approximate normal DL's.

Table 2 indicates the interpolated DL for each subject. These were obtained by interpolating between the judgments of the Δf immediately below the 70-percent judgment criterion and the Δf immediately above the criterion. The DL's are grouped into those presented above or equal to 1 KHz and those presented below or equal to 1 KHz, as well as by population.

The DL's obtained from retarded subjects were larger than those obtained from normal subjects for stimuli presented above the referent 1-KHz signal. One retarded subject, D. G., indicated a smaller DL than the largest normal-subject DL for stimuli presented below the referent 1-KHz signal. The mean retarded subject DL's were more than twice as large as the respective normal subject DL's for stimuli above and below the referent frequency of 1 KHz.

On the surface, the major difference between the normal and retarded subject DL's indicates that a retarded person cannot make frequency discriminations as fine as those made by a normal person. One could project this

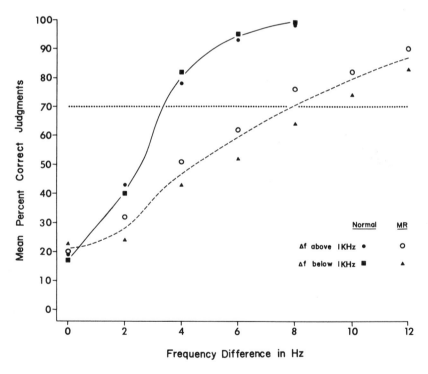

Figure 3. Percentage of correct judgments as a function of frequency difference (reference frequency = 1 KHz) for normal adults and severely retarded children. See text for detailed explanation.

Table 2. Individual subject and group interpolated DL's for all discriminative stimuli above and below the reference signal (1 KHz)

Subjects	Above 1 KHz	Below 1 KHz
Normal		
C. S.	5.1	4.5
C. D.	4.1	3.8
K. M.	1.3	2.4
F. S.	3.9	3.3
J. K.	2.7	2.6
	$\overline{X} = 3.4$	$\overline{X} = 3.3$
Retarded		
D. G.	7.2	3.9
D. H.	5.2	7.1
L. R.	6.5	10.8
B. H.	11.2	11.5
	$\overline{X} = 7.5$	$\overline{X} = 8.3$

deficiency into the speech domain and rationalize the difficulty that some retardates experience in perceiving speech. One also could postulate that the peripheral auditory system must not be the site of frequency DL judgments, inasmuch as retarded subjects with normal peripheral systems, i.e., on the basis of puretone thresholds, indicated high DL's.

However, these surface observations, assumptions, and projections do not give an accurate picture of the results in view of the procedures used with the two populations or in view of the results previously obtained by other investigators.

One need only look at the data of Riach (1967) and of Harris (1952) in Table 1 to notice that a given population can exhibit DL's over twice as large as those of another population, with all procedures and stimuli remaining constant. It is interesting to note that our four severely retarded subjects produced median DL's smaller than those of the high-school students in the study by Riach and that our five normal subjects produced median DL's smaller than those of the 20 university students in that study. The normal subjects in this study also produced smaller median DL's than those of Harris' subjects, who were not trained extensively.

It appears evident that the amount of training and experience acquired by subjects is as much a primary factor in determining DL size as is the population. Therefore, it cannot be stated unequivocally that the power of retarded subjects to resolve frequency is any less acute than that of normals.

It should be remembered that the procedural contingencies differed between populations in this study (the retarded subjects did not have a negative subtract contingency because of programming limitations). Within the normal population itself, there was considerable variability during pretraining sessions until an appropriate set of contingencies could be established; then variability decreased. The effects of differing contingency procedures are speculative.

From the data in this study, one cannot postulate that the retarded have more difficulty with speech and language than do normals because they cannot perceive the finite frequency changes required in the speech signal. Normal subject data compiled by Flanagan (1957) indicated that "... it should not be necessary to quantize formant frequency in steps smaller than about ± 20 cps for F1, ± 50 cps for F2, and ± 75 cps for F3." Both the second and third vowel formant can occur at approximately 1 KHz in the adult male phonation range. The retarded subjects in this study perceived frequency differences considerably smaller than those necessary for perceiving changes in these three vowel formants.

On the other hand, Martin, Pickett, and Colten (1972), investigating vowel formant transitions with severe sensorineural loss subjects, indicated that the ability to discriminate a primary formant frequency transition cue does not ensure speech perception. Often, the inclusion of low-frequency formant transitions tends to obscure the principal discrimination and to "reduce the ability to find these cues when they occur in a speech-like environment."

In summary, the modified method of the constant stimulus differences procedure is appropriate for obtaining frequency DL's, and the data are comparable with those of other studies. Although the DL's obtained from severely retarded subjects are larger than those obtained from the normal subjects, they fall within the limits of DL's obtained from minimally trained, normal-intelligence subjects.

LITERATURE CITED

Daniloff, R. G., T. J. Glattke, R. W. Keith, and A. M. Small, Jr. 1964. Procedural variables influencing estimations of different thresholds for frequency. J. Acoust. Soc. Amer. 36: 1733–1734.

Flanagan, J. L. 1957. Estimates of the maximum precision necessary in quantizing certain "dimensions" of vowel sounds. J. Acoust. Soc. Amer. 29: 533–534.

Flanagan, J. L., and M. G. Saslow. 1958. Pitch discrimination for synthetic vowels. J. Acoust. Soc. Amer. 30: 435–442.

Harris, J. D. 1948. Discrimination of pitch: Suggestions toward method and procedure. Amer. J. Psychol. 61: 309–322.

Harris, J. D. 1952. Pitch discrimination. J. Acoust. Soc. Amer. 24: 750–755.

Harris, J. D. 1969. Forty Germinal Papers in Human Hearing. The Journal of Auditory Research, Groton, Conn.

Henning, G. B. 1966. Frequency discrimination of random-amplitude tones. J. Acoust. Soc. Amer. 39: 336–339.

Lieberman, P. 1967. Intonation, Perception, and Language. (Research Monograph No. 38) The M.I.T. Press, Cambridge.

Martin, E. S., J. M. Pickett, and S. Colten. 1972. Discrimination of vowel formant transitions by listeners with severe sensorineural hearing loss. *In*: G. Fant (ed.), Proceedings of the International Symposium on Speech Communication Ability and Profound Deafness. The Alexander Graham Bell Association for the Deaf, Washington, D. C.

Michaels, R. M. 1957. Frequency difference limens for narrow bands of noise. J. Acoust. Soc. Amer. 29: 520–522.

Riach, W. D. 1967. Normative data on a battery of discrimination tests. *In*: A. B. Graham (ed.), Sensorineural Hearing Processes and Disorders, pp. 105–112. Little, Brown & Co., Boston.

Rosenblith, W. A., and K. N. Stevens. 1953. On the DL for frequency. J. Acoust. Soc. Amer. 25: 980–985.

Shower, E. G., and R. Biddulph. 1931. Differential pitch sensitivity of the ear. J. Acoust. Soc. Amer. 3: 275–287.

8 Detection of Intensity Increments

Robert T. Fulton and
Paul A. Waryas

We have discussed studies concerning two of the three basic parameters of all acoustic signals, duration and frequency. This chapter concerns intensity, the third basic parameter.

Since Riesz (see Harris, 1963) reported an amplitude modulation study over 40 years ago, intensity discrimination research has produced many pages of hard data, theoretical argument, clinical implications, and conflicting results. It is beyond the scope of this chapter to review all the pertinent literature. Readers are referred to Harris' monograph for a comprehensive review of procedures, theory, and clinical applications of intensity discrimination.

Few studies have been undertaken to relate intensity discrimination to the speech signal or to employ the speech signal as a discriminative stimulus. Flanagan (1972) reported three such studies. In one, the intensity DL for the second formant of the vowel /ae/ was found to be approximately 3 dB. A second study indicated a 1.5-dB DL for the overall intensity of a synthetic vowel. Since the first formant is usually the most intense formant in a vowel sound, Flanagan indicated that 1.5 dB might be a rough estimate of the first formant DL as well. A third study was directed at intensity DL's for single harmonic components of synthetic vowels. Flanagan indicated that DL's obtained at the first and second formant frequencies were commensurate with the 1.5- and 3.0-dB values mentioned above.

DIFFERENTIAL MEASURES WITH THE RETARDED

There are only three known studies in which an attempt was made to measure intensity DL's with the retarded (Dugas and Baumeister, 1968; Kopatic and Kopatic, 1969a, b).

Kopatic and Kopatic conducted three related experiments in an attempt to obtain reliable auditory (intensity) DL's with retarded subjects, mean age of 21.65 years and mean IQ of 60. The first experiment (1969a) used a method of limits procedure and obtained DL's (1.48 dB) less than one-half those obtained with a normal sample (3.39 dB), with constant errors of +1.93 and −0.33 dB, respectively. The investigators concluded that subsequent experiments were in order but that those experiments should use the method of constant stimuli and alter the duration between the two stimuli.

In the first of the next two experiments (Kopatic and Kopatic, 1969b), the only procedural alteration made was in the duration between stimuli. The same retarded persons as those previously examined were subjects in this experiment. Half of the subjects were presented with the stimuli 3 seconds apart and half 1 second apart. Reliability did not improve. In the final experiment, using the 10 most reliable subjects from the first two experiments, the procedure was changed to one of constant stimuli. Again, reliable results were not obtained and the investigators concluded that, "the results of this study and the one previously reported indicate that it is not possible to reliably examine auditory differential limens in the mentally handicapped using classical psychophysical methods."

Dugas and Baumeister (1968) investigated auditory DL variability as a result of distractors with retarded and normal subjects. The 18 retarded subjects had a mean age of 20.6 years and mean IQ of 64.8 (SD = 7.5). Subjects were required to indicate whether stimulus pairs were the same or different under three conditions of distraction: (a) light-off; (b) light-on; and (c) flashing light (a panel of lights was mounted in front of the subject). The DL was defined as half of the interval of uncertainty:

IU = Lu − L1. The Lu was defined as that point above standard intensity which was halfway between the first 'different' to 'same.' That point below standard intensity which was halfway between the last transition from 'same' to 'different' was defined as the L1.

Three blocks of DL's were administered in one day. Results indicated larger and more variable DL's with the retarded than with normals for all trials and for all distraction conditions. Mean DL's for the retarded ranged from 5.0 to 10.5 dB across trials and conditions. The intratrial variability of the retarded was evident across distractor conditions.

The subjects in the above experiments tended to be mildly to moderately retarded young adults. DL's were obtained statistically; stimulus differences were limited to 2-dB increments.

PURPOSE

The primary purpose of this study was to demonstrate the extension of the stimulus-response control paradigm to the investigation of differential intensity with difficult-to-test populations, specifically, the severely retarded.

METHOD

Subjects

Four severely retarded children, three males and one female, served as subjects for this study. Three subjects (D. H., D. G., and L. R.) had taken part in both of the previous psychoacoustic studies, i.e., duration and frequency. The fourth subject (T. P.) had participated in the duration study. Subject IQ's ranged from 29 to 40, and chronological ages, from 12 to 17 years.

Subject Selection Criteria

Each subject was required to meet a two-phase pretest criterion before the experimental program was begun. Phase 1 consisted of obtaining an operant puretone threshold average (three sessions at 1 KHz) within normal limits. Phase 2 consisted of meeting an 18/20 criterion (at least 18 correct responses to 20 consecutive stimuli) to pretest stimuli for three consecutive 20-stimulus blocks. The pretest stimuli were 250-millisecond[1], 5-dB intensity increments superimposed on a 20-dB SL, 1-KHz continuous pedestal signal. The auditory stimulus conditions were designed to be acoustically similar to the conditions found in the SISI test. The signals were presented on a VI 10-second schedule. A probability generator controlled presentation of test stimuli (70-percent probability) or nonincrement control stimuli (30-percent probability). Between two and eight three-block sessions were required for subjects to meet the pretest criterion. It was determined that this relatively strict criterion was necessary to ensure subject stimulus-response control.

---

[1] The instrumentation was set to generate the duration of the SISI signal recommended by Harford (1967): 200 milliseconds peak-to-peak, with 50-millisecond rise-and-fall times. Using photographic oscilloscope analyses of the actual signal and the formula of Dallos and Olsen (1964) ($T = 2/3r + P$) for equivalent durations, we found the signal to be 250 milliseconds. The perfect signal according to the recommendation of Harford and the formula of Dallos and Olsen would be 266.6 milliseconds in equivalent duration.

Instrumentation

All sessions were conducted in a sound-treated room (Industrial Acoustics Co.). An audio oscillator (Hewlett-Packard Model 201CR) generated both the 1-KHz continuous pedestal tone and the pedestal tone increments. The oscillator output was divided between two attenuator systems (Hewlett-Packard Model 350D) mixed by a two-channel speech audiometer (Grason-Stadler Model 162) and routed to a 10-ohm button-type audioreceiver (Dyna Magnetic Devices, Model D308). The receiver was kept in place in right ears by custom earmolds. Dummy receivers and earmolds were placed in the left ears of the subjects.

The block diagram of the instrumentation is the same as that for the short-duration study (Chapter 6, Figure 2) except that a third custom-made attenuator was connected in series with Attenuator B. A detailed schematic of the programming instrumentation may be found in Appendix G. Special notice should be taken of the two attenuation systems. Attenuation System A controlled the pedestal tone. The electronic switch remained on continuously, and the attenuator (Hewlett-Packard Model 350D), in conjunction with the black channel of the speech audiometer, controlled the intensity of the pedestal tone. Attenuator System B (a Hewlett-Packard Model 350D and the custom-made attenuator) controlled the pedestal increments. The electronic switch was set for 50-millisecond rise-and-fall times and was programmed for an "on" time of 200 milliseconds on a VI 10-second schedule. Summation of the two intensities in the speech audiometer produced an output approximately 6 dB above the continuous 1-KHz pedestal. The custom-made attenuator, in series with a second standard attenuator (Hewlett-Packard Model 350D), controlled the intensity of the pedestal increment. The custom attenuator was adjusted for intensity increments of 5.0, 1.4, 1.2, 1.0, 0.8, and 0.6 dB on a Bruel and Kjaer Type 2203 sound-level meter (A scale). A 0.0-dB increment in the pedestal tone was obtained by adjusting the Hewlett-Packard attenuator for 50 dB of attenuation, more than was necessary for functional removal of Attenuator System B from audibility. All of the attenuator settings were controlled manually. The response circuit predelay was set for 300 milliseconds and the postdelay was set for 2.0 seconds. Intertrial responses (ITR's) resulted in a 5-second time out. Reinforcement was provided on a FR-3 reinforcement ratio for correct stimulus detection, i.e., every third correct-button response by subjects resulted in the delivery of a reinforcer. Every correct response was reinforced by a door chime within the reinforcement delivery apparatus.

Procedure

At the beginning of each test session, the 1-KHz pedestal tone was presented at 20 dB above the mean threshold of each subject. Subjects were required to meet a 9/10 pretest criterion, i.e., to respond correctly to nine of 10 consecutive 5-dB increment presentations in the 20-dB SL pedestal. The 5-dB increments were programmed by probability along with zero-dB control increments, i.e., each 5-dB increment had a 70-percent chance of occurring and each zero-dB increment had a 30-percent chance of occurring. The pretest criterion phase was established to determine whether subjects were under stimulus-response control at the start of each test session.

The experimental test session consisted of a 20-dB SL pedestal signal and the random delivery of 70 stimulus increments, 10 presentations each of 5.0-, 1.4-, 1.2-, 1.0-, 0.8-, 0.6-, and 0.0-dB increments. The 5.0- and 0.0-dB increments served as controls for subject under- and overresponding, respectively. Because the 0.0-dB increment was included in the stimulus group, the probability of occurrence was set for 100 percent during the experimental conditions. The stimulus increments were controlled manually but were delivered automatically on a predetermined random schedule. Individual event responses were recorded manually. Electromechanical counters recorded totals of the number of stimuli presented, the number of correct responses, the ITR's, and the total number of subject responses for each session. Three blocks of 10 sessions constituted the experimental program.

RESULTS AND DISCUSSION

The mean percentage of intensity-increment detections by subject and session block are found in Table 1. One of the four subjects (T. P.) was unable to meet Phase 2 (18 correct responses to 20 consecutive pretest stimuli) and therefore did not receive the experimental stimuli.

The results of the completion of all experimental sessions by the three subjects indicate:

1. Only one subject (D. H.) demonstrated a DL_{50} with the intensity increments under investigation, and the 50-percent level was not attained until the third block of sessions.
2. Only one subject (D. H.) demonstrated detection rates above 20 percent for the 1.0-dB increment (20 percent is the upper limit for negative results with the SISI).
3. There was a tendency for a slight increase in detection rate by session block means, indicating some practice effects. However, these increases

Table 1. Mean percentage of detections (relative to 20 dB SL) per intensity increment (N = 100; 10 trials per session, 10 sessions per mean) by subject and session block

Subject	Sessions	Intensity increments (relative to 20 dB SL pedestal)						
		0*	0.6	0.8	1.0	1.2	1.4	5.0*
D. H.	1–10	08	09	14	26	33	46	91
	11–20	05	09	15	22	23	48	85
	21–30	11	18	33	38	50	64	92
L. R.	1–10	00	03	01	04	03	11	67
	11–20	05	03	08	05	05	12	67
	21–30	03	03	07	10	10	16	85
D. G.	1–10	04	07	07	05	13	26	80
	11–20	09	13	15	10	14	25	87
	21–30	04	04	05	18	13	35	93

*Controls.

were not consistent and not of the magnitude found in the SISI experiments (see Chapter 4).

The results are not as definitive as one might hope for discussion; however, they do suggest some issues. Intrasubject detection rates were highly variable between sessions and session blocks. Intrasubject variability is common with retarded children, particularly those with low intellectual and functional capabilities. However, the means of session blocks per increment, representing 100 trials for each (10 trials per session, 10 sessions per block), are reasonably similar.

The subject (D. H.) indicating the highest detection rates also indicated the highest rate of responses to the 0.0-dB control period. The subject (L. R.) with the best record for not responding to the 0.0-dB control period also had the poorest detection rate for the increments. These data illustrate subjects who select individual likelihood ratio strategies. (Green and Swets, 1966)

The effects of practice were not as evident in this experiment as had been indicated by some subjects in the SISI experiments. This decline may be due to the fact that the subjects in this experiment might be classified as "experienced listeners," in view of their practice in the duration and frequency discrimination tests.

The primary purpose of demonstrating the extension of the stimulus-response control model to the investigation of differential intensity was achieved. However, other than for D. H., the resulting data did not produce individual intensity DL_{50}, as had been hoped. As a result of subsequent modifications, i.e., raising the pedestal signal to 35 dB SL and increasing each intensity increment by 1 dB (1.6–2.4 instead of 0.6–1.4), two additional subjects (L. R. and D. G.) provided DL_{50} (number of trials = 100) at the 1.8-dB increment. T. P. (the subject who was unable to meet original pretest criteria) increased her detection rate but failed to achieve a level of 50-percent detection even at the 2.4-dB increment.

To illustrate further the applicability of the stimulus-response control intensity-detection model, we subsequently conducted an additional two-phase experiment. The first phase was designed to investigate intensity-increment performance as a function of sound pressure level in relation to equal perceptual levels between subjects. The first condition was a replication of the experiment reported above, that is, the pedestal was presented at 20 dB SL. In the second condition, we introduced narrow-band noise ipsilaterally until the threshold was raised 20 dB and then added the 20-dB base pedestal above that threshold. The third condition followed the same procedure as the second, except that narrow-band noise was inserted until the threshold was raised 40 dB. The results were variable but tended to indicate, as anticipated, that intensity-detection performance increases as sound pressure level is increased.

In the second phase, we examined intensity-increment detection performance as a function of signal-to-noise levels. Again, the results were highly variable but indicated, as anticipated, that detection performance increased as the signal-to-noise levels increased.

The results of the experiments conducted subsequent to the initial experiment are not significant in terms of providing normative data with the retarded. This is true even with the initial experiment. The data do suggest, however, that severely retarded children do not differ grossly from normals in intensity-increment detection and that this performance is related to the intensity of the presentation level, as it is with normals.

What is significant, however, is the demonstration that the stimulus-response control paradigm is applicable to the investigation of the intensity parameter with difficult-to-test populations, specifically, to the severely retarded. Furthermore, it demonstrates that severely retarded children, at least in the sample used, are capable of processing simple signals in the presence of a competing complex signal (narrow-band noise) presented ipsilaterally. This latter factor is particularly significant in view of the folk beliefs that the retarded are incapable of responding to abstract auditory signals and that it is not possible to use classical psychophysical methods to examine auditory functions with the retarded.

LITERATURE CITED

Dallos, P. J., and W. O. Olsen. 1964. Integration of energy at threshold with gradual rise-fall tone pips. J. Acoust. Soc. Amer. 36: 743–751.

Dugas, J. L., and A. A. Baumeister. 1968. A comparison of intra-subject variability in auditory difference limens of normals and retardates. Amer. J. Ment. Defic. 73: 500–504.

Flanagan, J. L. 1972. Speech Analysis Synthesis and Perception, 2nd Ed. Springer-Verlag, New York.

Green, D. M., and J. A. Swets. 1966. Signal Detection Theory and Psychophysics, John Wiley & Sons, Inc., New York.

Harford, E. 1967. Clinical application and significance of the SISI test. *In:* A. B. Graham (ed.), Sensorineural Hearing Processes and Disorders, pp. 223–233. Little, Brown & Co., Boston.

Harris, J. D. 1963. Loudness discrimination. J. Speech Hear. Dis. Monogr. Suppl. No. 11.

Kopatic, N. J., and N. Kopatic. 1969a. The reliability of mental retardates in judging subjective phenomena. Train. Sch. Bull. 65: 126–129.

Kopatic, N. J., and N. Kopatic. 1969b. The reliability of mental retardates in judging subjective phenomena. Part II. Train. Sch. Bull. 66: 86–88.

Overview
and Implications

Overview
and Implications

The application of the operant paradigm, stimulus → response → consequence, to evaluation of the hearing of behaviorally difficult populations is not new. Many researchers and clinicians have applied the principles in various forms, generally manipulating the reinforcing agent. However, few have approached the problems of contingency management in a systematic manner. Therefore, it is understandable that many have been disappointed by their first experience with this approach. Some even have rejected the principles.

We have attempted to show that these principles generally are applicable to the problems of auditory measurement with difficult-to-test populations. The training procedures outlined and discussed in Chapter 1 were designed and modified, yet remain subject to continued modification, on the premise that a universal training procedure is applicable and efficient for audiometric test battery applications. More specifically, if a subject is systematically trained to respond to a basic "core" system, i.e., if he is brought under stimulus-response control, a variety of tests then can be administered with minimal adjustment. In essence, the difficult-to-test child is taught to respond to changes in his auditory environment. Test application then is merely a task of arranging the discriminative stimuli in a manner which best utilizes this skill.

Three audiologic test procedures, puretone thresholds, SISI, and threshold tone decay, have been demonstrated to be adaptable to a basic operant discrimination (detection) model. All three procedures are modeled around a singular paradigm, thus permitting rapid generalization between procedures. As a result of varying degrees of experience and application, the procedures reflect varying degrees of refinement.

The puretone threshold procedure has received substantial support through tests of reliability and efficacy of application. The tone decay procedure was the latest to be developed, and thus its utility remains to be determined. The SISI procedure is somewhere in between, with some degree of uncertainty because of the demonstration of practice influences.

The inclusion of these three tests by no means indicates that these are the only tests, or for that matter the preferred ones, to be included in a test battery. As indicated, the validity of the SISI test is questionable by any procedure, whether operant or standard handraising. In many clinics, impedance audiometry has superseded bone-conduction thresholds. We prefer impedance measurements in our own clinical practice. However, we have not abandoned bone-conduction totally because it serves as an intertest validation measure.

The significance of the research thus far is that the principles and the concept are sound and that this approach provides a substantial contribution to solving the problem of audiologic assessment with the difficult-to-test.

Despite the obvious need for continued investigation, the significant factor arising from the audiologic research conducted thus far is that definitive results can be obtained with difficult-to-test populations. It is also significant to note that the hearing of persons heretofore relegated to gross assessments may be assessed with greater confidence and finesse.

The section on psychoacoustics illustrates the generalized application of the principles to the investigation of basic acoustics. The presentation of research with the parameters of time, frequency, and intensity are only illustrative of the auditory research which can be conducted with difficult-to-test individuals; the potential for research in this area is virtually unlimited. Again, the basic stimulus-response-consequence model remains intact and basically the same throughout these investigations. The subjects used in the psychoacoustic studies were trained, thresholds were obtained, and the experiments were conducted using the same basic response, programming and stimulus generation and control apparatus.

The three psychoacoustic parameters, duration, frequency, and intensity, that were investigated in Chapters 6–8 were limited to the detection of simple signals. However, the results indicate that the severely retarded children in these studies are capable of responding to these parameters in a manner not grossly different from that of normal adults. It was also demonstrated that they are capable of discriminating simple signals at levels which are relevant to speech perception.

However, we are not suggesting a broad set of theoretical implications for speech perception. At this juncture, nothing is known about the skill of the retardate in integrating and processing the interactions of these variables.

In summary, this line of research, based on the $S^D \rightarrow R \rightarrow S^R$ paradigm, indicates that:

1. An audiometric assessment battery for the difficult-to-test is feasible and can be developed around a universal response model, eliminating the problem of diverse and complex instructions.
2. Difficult-to-test children, specifically the severely retarded, can be assessed by air- and bone-conduction threshold, short-increment sensitivity index, and threshold tone decay audiometric procedures. Several of these procedures have been applied to other difficult-to-test populations.
3. The training of basic auditory discriminative principles is similar to the training of basic concepts, which generalize across discrimination tasks.
4. Severely retarded children can provide reliable intersession response data.
5. Severely retarded children can respond to finite auditory discrimination tasks in a manner similar to that of normal adults, according to central tendency data; however, retardates show a slightly larger response variability.
6. Severely retarded children can discriminate individual acoustic parameters of duration, frequency, and intensity to a finer degree than is necessary for the perception of speech stimuli.

More important than the data themselves are two major issues and/or areas of systematic research: first, the opening of new auditory-response control investigative areas, and second, the introduction of assessment procedures with implications for amelioration for the difficult-to-test.

Procedural applications to a variety of problems were presented and discussed. These were presented to illustrate how the principles can be applied to both clinical and basic research. The model and the procedures described are not a panacea, nor are they beyond reproach. In addition, they will not solve all behavioral problems with the difficult-to-test. At the time of application, we felt that these procedures were the most appropriate for our goals; however, they do not constitute the ultimate approach. There is still a need for refined and improved procedures.

Research may lead to additional modifications in the training procedures, which may be the first formal and comprehensive learning models for many subjects with severe behavioral problems. That is, this may be their first experience with a task in which they understand the rules and consequences. If this is true, then such a program may be basic to training in all forms of communication requiring an auditory stimulus. Also, a child who finds a system in which he can succeed will be more *motivated, intrigued,* and *attentive* and will be more likely to succeed on subsequent tasks. The overall effect can be a decrease in disruptive behaviors and increased response rates that would seem to indicate heightened motivation.

All of these factors are relevant to subsequent training, and this fact alone may be the big bonus from this procedural model. Without shortchanging its significance, except as a reference, one should keep in mind the fact that the attainment of a screening test or puretone threshold may be inconsequential in comparison with the development of a total training framework. As in nursery school or kindergarten, it may be more important for a child to develop functional relationships than it is for him to accomplish a specific semirelated task. With children who are developmentally or mentally retarded, it is obvious that extensive corrective programs are needed to develop frameworks on which programs can be presented. It is conceded that the initial time required to complete the training phases may exceed that of the time required to use some other behavioral system, such as "block dropping"; nevertheless, the generalization potential of the proposed training program is much greater.

The data indicate that the retarded are more variable in their response behaviors than are normal adult populations. However, central tendency mean data are reasonably similar. There is a tendency for intrasession variability with retarded subjects. For the most part, the experiments presented in this book were not designed to control for this variability and therefore are subject to this criticism.

Intrasession variability suggests that intrasession control stimuli should be presented to the subject. These control stimuli would be those which the examiner knows the subject can easily detect. If the subject fails to respond to a substantial percentage of these control stimuli during a session, that session or the appropriate portion of it would be excluded from the data. This procedure probably would result in the exclusion of parts of sessions in which control is lost temporarily because of satiation, petit mal seizure, or other factors. Pilot work to control this type of response behavior has been conducted. The results were inconclusive in that different behaviors were indicated by the subjects involved. Nevertheless, the problem remains; thus, the area of intrasession control needs more investigation and clarification.

The continuous presence of this issue is highly supportive of the position that subject control is as critical as stimulus control, a point seldom alluded to in auditory research. That is, as much emphasis should be placed on the control of subject response behavior as on the control of the stimulus with which the subject is presented. The lack of attention to both areas of control is evidenced throughout our history by the constant referral to the inability of subjects to respond to traditional procedures. Consequently, procedures usually are "watered down" or discarded. That is, we present stimuli of unknown or assumed characteristics because they appear to result in more easily obtainable responses than do controlled and/or more desirable stimuli, or we accept responses of questionable reliability. The *procedure* fails more often than does the *child*.

Throughout this book, there has been repeated discussion of the generalization of the principles of response behavior between tasks. It was implied that once a child has developed a specific response behavior, it has broad general application. As empirical and clinical as it may be, the following case report may exemplify the generalization of this principle between unrelated tasks.

J. E. is a nonverbal, severely retarded girl (age 8 years, 9 months; SQ, 25). She was selected as a subject for a nonverbal language concept development program in order to determine whether she could be trained to conceptualize a complex language structure by a symbolic nonspeech response mode (Carrier, in press; Premack, 1970). J. E.'s entry behavior—inattentive, unwilling to accept reinforcement, unstimulated by language form blocks, and generally ill-behaved—was sufficiently disturbing that, after 37 sessions, no significant progress had been made, even in behavior control. After one short-term attempt, approximately 1 year before the nonverbal language program, an operant puretone threshold assessment had been terminated for lack of behavior control.

We decided that perhaps J. E. had not acquired the concept of learning, or of discriminative response and its related facets. Therefore, we began a concerted effort to complete a "by-the-book" operant puretone threshold with J. E. The basic training procedures used in the puretone test procedure are analogous to the concept of discriminative learning.

Initial puretone stimulus-response training sessions were as unsuccessful as had been the initial language training sessions, i.e., the subject sat and did nothing. It required 12 sessions before J. E. completed Phase 1 (button response to an auditory signal) of the stimulus-response control procedures. There was a gradual improvement in J. E.'s response behavior. After a total of 25 sessions, the subject met stimulus-response pretraining criteria and was ready for threshold assessment. Air- and bone-conduction thresholds were obtained, double-checked by a second examiner, and found to be reliable (± 5 dB). By this time, the subject's overall behavior had changed. She was attentive, consumed edible reinforcers, and indicated a discriminative response pattern (low intertrial and control responses).

Pretraining phases (Phases 2–10) were rerun, after threshold assessment, to check for differences in response patterns. J. E. completed all phases in one session lasting 29 minutes, 54 seconds, whereas the initial training period had taken 25 sessions of 9 hours, 52 minutes, 16 seconds.

J. E. was returned to the aforementioned language training program, where she immediately responded as an attentive, discriminative subject. Her progress in the language training program has continued.

This case study is not intended to imply a cure-all for all behavioral ills. In fact, it is possible that improvement in both tasks was due to a third, unknown, factor. However, this case and other examples have caused us to consider that many of the principles encompassed by the pretraining stimulus-response control procedures are applicable to subsequent training programs.

The psychoacoustics research thus far conducted has been limited to the detection of simple signals. Even this research needs considerable broadening, e.g., there should be investigation of frequency DL's at frequencies other than 1 KHz and of the effects of various stimulus rise-and-fall times. Considerable procedural research needs to be conducted, e.g., into the use of intrasession controls to reduce subject variability. No research has been conducted on the interaction of the three basic parameters (duration, frequency, and intensity) investigated herein.

Little research has been conducted on the effects of signal discrimination in the presence of interference. This area is significant with difficult-to-test populations because in such cases the task becomes one of processing rather than of simple detection or discrimination. This area introduces new variables of binaural hearing and ipsilateral and contralateral interference. Beyond this is the area of binaural integration, which includes filtered and temporal interrupted signals.

These areas feed into the broad area of speech perception, with its interaction of psychoacoustic and speech variables, the latter including both real and artificial stimuli.

The investigation of speech perception from a purely acoustic base should shed considerable light on the problem of auditory perception, which in turn is crucial to the processes of learning and amelioration.

With this in mind, studies of more complex discriminations such as formant transitions, speech-versus-nonspeech stimuli, binaural discriminations, distortion, and auditory memory are appropriate. A continuing effort should be directed toward attempts to find an auditory perceptual breakdown, if one is present. The experience that we gain in assessing these functions will be valuable in later development of ameliorative programs. In fact, these areas should be investigated simultaneously, thus providing each other with the appropriate feedback.

The psychoacoustic and speech perception work also can provide significant input into the continued development of audiologic test development. The investigation of psychoacoustic parameters which are similar to those in audiologic tests provides information in dual areas. Research into the areas of signal integration and speech perception has potential for the development of central audiologic assessment tools.

The psychoacoustic section has attempted to open an exciting new area of research. However, the discriminative response relationships to specific language functions with developmentally limited populations need to be investigated thoroughly before the development of relevant and efficient communication training programs can be completed. This fact should not preclude the planning, piloting, and probing of procedures for advancing the process of amelioration.

It seems appropriate to postulate that, in general, the retarded are not restricted by an inherent inability to discriminate perceptually, although many may be deficient in strategy and concept skills for processing complex auditory signals. It therefore may be necessary to establish a conceptual framework or set of rules and principles on which retardates can base their subsequent processing training and experience. There are rules and concepts which must be firmly affixed before an individual can deal appropriately with language. Therefore, a similar set of rules and concepts may be necessary for auditory perception.

If such a premise is valid, then it is essential to identify the rules and principles underlying the development of auditory perception skills.

Our initial and current thoughts in this direction center on three basic auditory processing principles and their related, but generalized, approaches:

Concept	Task
The environment is composed of auditory changes	Train subjects to respond to the detection of auditory changes (detection)
Differential auditory stimuli have "associative" meaning	Train subjects to respond differentially to auditory stimuli (discrimination)
Auditory stimuli can be lawfully processed and classified	Train subjects to generalize their responses to functional classes (categorization)

The model presented and discussed throughout this work has been directed toward the process of detection, as opposed to discrimination and categorization. However, that does not preclude the extension of behavioral control principles to the other areas. In fact, it adds support to the contention that the principles are equally as relevant to training as they are to assessment.

In view of what is known and what has been postulated, there are two potential research strategies. One is to proceed slowly, carefully investigating the boundaries of each parameter to insure against pitfalls. The other strategy is to leap forward, assuming that a general knowledge of the overall problem is more significant than detailed knowledge of a portion of that problem. Both strategies have merit and should be pursued. The first is subject to the criticism of "dragging its feet" on a problem requiring "long overdue" amelioration and applied relevance. The second can be criticized because it may overrun its interference or tactical support and jeopardize the basic strength of the attack. Also, with the second strategy, there is the possibility of prostituting research integrity.

The first strategy is individually the safest, while the second is more exciting. With these problems in mind, we have decided to try to walk the fine line between the advantages of speedy research and the requirements for sound research, hoping for the excitement of looking into new areas while closing the gaps, as best we can, on critical variables along the way.

In conjunction with the research strategies selected is our view that the study of inoperative systems, whether they are behaviorally oriented or physiologic, is the best avenue for gaining increased knowledge about the function of that system. We believe that we can learn more about the communication process from persons with inoperative systems than from persons with intact systems. If such a premise is true, then there is a multitude of populations available and willing to assist us as subjects in our search for increased knowledge about man's most important function, communication.

The three main goals of this work have been attained: (a) we have described the mechanics and procedures for assessing difficult-to-test individuals, (b) we have demonstrated procedural applications to both clinical and basic auditory assessment, and (c) we have provided data which are useful for a better understanding of the auditory functioning of retarded children and information which can be used to develop programs for training communication skills.

The research reported herein should not be construed as the completion of auditory discrimination research with the retarded or the difficult-to-test or as defining the limitations of the stimulus-response control model proposed. If anything, it reflects only a beginning.

This work itself imposes the same dimensions of development as does the content of the material. That is, there is no conceivable way to transmit all of the information which has been accumulated or the experiences which have been encountered. We can hope only to have imparted the basic principles to the reader; it then becomes his responsibility to generalize the principles through additional experiences. The effort expended by the reader through experiences will broaden and strengthen this knowledge, as demonstrated by the subjects in their experiences.

The implications of this entire line of research and the use of this model go far beyond the needs of the developmentally disabled. The results of such investigations will contribute to the auditory assessment of many persons who for various reasons are difficult-to-test.

LITERATURE CITED

Carrier, J. K., Jr. Application of functional analysis and a non-speech response mode to teaching language. *In* L. McReynolds (ed.), Developing Systematic Procedures for Training Children Language. ASHA Monograph No. 18 (In press)

Premack, D. 1970. A functional analysis of language. J. Exp. Anal. Behav. 14: 107–125.

Appendices

A Detailed Procedures for Training Auditory Stimulus-Response Control and for Obtaining Audiometric Puretone Thresholds

Robert T. Fulton
and
Joseph E. Spradlin

INTRODUCTION

The following audiologic test procedures were designed to be used with mentally retarded and other difficult-to-test persons, and to be operative with the Allison 22 audiometer and the electromechanical relay programming system described in Appendices B and C.

Reinforcer

An effective reinforcer should be determined prior to the beginning of the training. The subject will tell the examiner, in a variety of ways, which reinforcer is good. If the reinforcing event is nutritive, the child may open his mouth or stick out his tongue when the nutritive is placed near his mouth. If the event is social, the subject may smile or laugh or attempt to hold the examiner's hand. A reinforcing event is anything that a specific child will work to obtain.

Earphone Placement

After the child is seated in the experimental room, the earphones are put in place. Many difficult-to-test children will allow the earphones to be placed in position and will not attempt to remove them. In this case, the examiner should proceed directly to the training program.

If the child refuses the earphones initially, several techniques can be used to train him to wear them. The examiner may choose to deliver reinforcement contingent on the child's allowing the earphones to be brought closer and closer to position. Such successive approximation training usually is effective but often slow.

A second, less desirable, procedure is simply to position the earphones and hold them in place, applying pressure with the thumbs behind the child's ears for as long as he struggles. When the child relaxes, pressure is removed. If the child begins to struggle again, pressure is reinstated. The procedure is not elegant, but it usually is effective. During this procedure, the examiner may choose to deliver positive reinforcement when the child is not resisting. This may speed the training process for two reasons: first, reaching for reinforcement is somewhat incompatible with resisting earphones; and second, ceasing to resist is reinforced by release of pressure and by positive reinforcers.

Once the child is wearing the earphones, the experimenter trains the subject to respond by presenting the tone to him and demonstrating the response. After each demonstration, the child is reinforced. After a couple of demonstrations, the examiner takes the child's hand and moves it through the response pattern while the tone is present. The child is reinforced. After two or three such aided responses, the child often can perform the response by himself. If the child does not respond independently after 10 or 12 aided trials, it may be necessary to use a "shaping" procedure in which the examiner assists the subject through successive approximations in response behavior.

Response Button

The response button requires a downward pressure for activation. A light, mounted under the Plexiglas and perforated steel response button, may be used as a visual cue to the physical location of the response button. Most subjects do not require the use of the light, and the absence of a light does not prolong training.

Once the child responds independently, the following automatic training program is instituted.

INITIAL AUTOMATIC PROGRAM FOR TRAINING

Training is intended to establish a response to a change in the auditory signal as a discriminative stimulus (S^D), rather than to establish a response to the simple presence of a tone. This technique is used because later stages of hearing testing often require the child to respond to a change in tone intensity or to a tone superimposed on a background signal, i.e., masking or pedestal tone.

Ambient Noise

A background of controlled ambient noise is used. The subject is trained to respond to discriminative stimuli which differ in intensity and/or frequency. These discriminations often are needed later in the masking of unilateral air-conduction losses or bone-conduction thresholds. Intensity discrimination in the presence of a pedestal tone is required for the short-increment sensitivity index (SISI). Training the subject to respond to acoustic changes in the ambient noise from the "outset" is easier than "fading in" the necessary background signals at a later date. Once the subject has been trained to respond differentially, the background signal can be eliminated for threshold measurements with no adverse effects.

Narrow-band masking centered on 750 Hz is used initially as a background signal (neutral stimulus). The masking signal is presented at an intensity above threshold and approximately 20–30 dB below the peak intensity of the S^D. (Narrow-band filters reduce the mean power of white noise by approximately 20 dB. A system for obtaining appropriate masking levels with the Allison 22 audiometer and Model 25 filter is as follows: insert white noise into Channel 2, calibrating the signal with the filter in the "out" position, on the VU meter; adjust the Channel 2 attenuator to the same level as the test signal—Channel 1—and then turn the filter to "in." The masking level will be approximately 20 dB below the peak intensity for the S^D.) The ambient noise background is presented binaurally until later phases in the training program.

Test Signal (S^D)

A 500-Hz tone 5 seconds in duration is used as the initial S^D. The S^D is presented at 30 dB above the estimated threshold of the subject or at 70 dB relative to audiometric zero. A more intense tone may be required if the subject is thought to have a significant hearing loss. A 500-Hz signal has been found to be pleasant and sensitive to most subjects. (In the automated program, the test signal is presented through Channel 1.)

Test Signal (S^D) Parameters

The S^D duration (5 seconds) is controlled by a timer. A reinforcer is delivered if the subject responds during the S^D period. In order to prevent reinforcement of "chance" responses made simultaneously with the onset of the S^D (the S^D would not be audible to the subject), a predelay timer delays the activation of the response circuit by 300 milliseconds. Also, to prevent the nonreinforcement of responses made simultaneously with the termination of the S^D (the termination of the S^D would not be apparent), a postdelay timer delays the termination of the response circuit by 300 milliseconds. That is to say that the response circuit remains open for the same duration as the S^D but is shifted 300 milliseconds later in time. The test signal is presented binaurally until later in the training program.

Control Periods

Nonaudible periods with the same temporal characteristics as those of the S^D are alternated by 50-percent duty cycle with the S^D. The use of control periods provides a systematic check on whether the responses of the subject are discriminative or attributable to chance. Steppers or probability generators can be used to program a random presentation of S^D's and controls.

Presentation of S^D and Control Periods

The alternating S^D and control periods are presented on a variable interval of 6 seconds. That is, the periods are initiated on the average of one each 6 seconds, with variable intervals between presentations. VI schedules help to prevent the subject from responding to a fixed interval of time.

Intertrial Interval and Responses

The intervals between S^D and control periods are called the intertrial intervals (ITI's). Responses made during an ITI result in a 5-second time out, a period during which the program is inoperative and, consequently, during which reinforcement cannot be earned.

A stainless-steel plate surrounds the response button and a perforated steel plate is embedded in it; these are the touch plates. Bodily contact with these metal plates triggers a capacitance device, which in turn initiates a time out (time out begins when contact is broken). The touch plate prevents the subject from fumbling or playing with the response mechanism when a trial is about to be presented; with the touch plate, a trial cannot be presented until 5 seconds after termination of the contact. Trained responses thereby become discrete responses and seldom are associated with accidental touching or random playing with the response button.

Response Control Criteria

The determination of whether a subject is under stimulus-response control is determined by recording his responses to S^D and control periods. If the subject responds randomly, a significant percentage of the responses will occur during the control periods. However, if he is discriminative, he will respond during S^D periods and refrain from responding during control periods. Subjects are required to meet response-control criteria for each phase before proceeding to the next phase. "Response criterion" is defined as response to all S^D periods with no responses during control periods for five consecutive and alternating pairs of presentations (5/0), unless otherwise specified.

The program is established as described above and remains in effect until changes are specified in the detailed phases stated below.

Training Phases

Phase 1. Initiate Response Topography
Criterion: obtain a subjective evaluation of response control, disregarding responses to control periods until the subject appears to be under control.

Phase 2. Response Control
Continue with the same program as Phase 1, but now evaluate responses to control periods (50-percent, alternating duty cycle for S^D and controls).
Criterion: response control criterion (5/0).

Phase 3. Signal Duration (3 Seconds)
Reduce S^D interval to 3 seconds.
Criterion: response control criterion (5/0).

Phase 4. Signal Duration (2 Seconds)
Reduce S^D interval to 2 seconds.
Criterion: response control criterion (5/0).

Phase 5. Environmental Stimulus Generalization (Noise)
Generalize the narrow-band ambient noise (750 Hz) to adjacent noise bands centered on 1 KHz and 500 Hz, maintaining intensity above threshold levels and 20–30 dB below the S^D intensity or intensities, as described in the program.

Criterion: response control criterion (5/0) for each band (return to successful bands as required to assist in generalization).

Phase 6. Environmental Stimulus Generalization (Puretone)
Generalize from noise bands to pedestal-puretone frequencies (order 1 KHz, 750 Hz, 500 Hz), maintaining pedestal intensity at 10 dB relative to estimated threshold.
Criterion: response control criterion (5/0) for each pedestal frequency (return to successful pedestals as required to assist in generalization).

Phase 7. Fading-out Environmental Stimulus
Fade out 500-Hz background signal (last background signal used in Phase 6) in 10-dB increments for each two consecutive, correct responses.
Maintain S^D at 30 dB relative to estimated threshold.
Criterion: response control criterion (5/0) after ambient-noise level has been faded out.

Phase 8. Discriminative Stimulus Generalization
Generalize S^D to other frequencies (order 500 Hz, 1 KHz, 2 KHz, 4 KHz, 8 KHz, 2 KHz, 500 Hz, and 250 Hz).
Criterion: two consecutive responses (2/0) at each frequency before proceeding to next frequency. If the subject misses two consecutive responses, return to a previously successful frequency for two responses, then try generalization again.

Phase 9. Stimulus Intensity Generalization
Reduce S^D (500-Hz) intensity in 20-dB increments until control is lost or intensity has been reduced to near screening levels. Repeat at 1 KHz.
Criterion: two consecutive responses at each intensity level.

Phase 10. Unilateral Generalization
Unilaterally present 500 Hz S^D at 20–30 dB relative to estimated threshold.
Criterion: response control criterion (5/0) for each ear.

Assessment Phases

Phase 11. Threshold (or Screening) Assessment
Criterion before assessment: the subject must meet response control, at suprathreshold levels, in *each session* before any threshold or screening measures are obtained for that session. (Criterion: respond to nine of 10

signal presentations and to no more than one of 10 controls for 10 consecutive and alternating pairs of events.)

Screening Program The subject is assessed for octave frequencies (250 Hz to 8 KHz bilaterally) at 1969 American National Standards Institute (ANSI) or 1964 ISO levels. If the subject fails two or more frequencies for either ear, then he fails screening criteria, and all frequencies are assessed according to the threshold program.

Threshold Program. Assess thresholds by the descending schedule of Carhart and Jerger (1959). "Threshold" is defined as the lowest intensity level at which the subject maintains a 50-percent response rate for a minimum of six trials for that level. Assess bone-conduction thresholds in a manner similar to that for air-conduction thresholds. Masking procedures are applied in accordance with rules established by Studebaker (1964).

Masking Procedure

Phases 12–14 are intended only for pretraining and adaptation and should not be interpreted as correct masking procedures, inasmuch as the subject already has had previous training in detecting the discriminative stimulus from environmental stimuli.

Phase 12.
Present 500-Hz S^D (automatic, 2 seconds, with controls, VI-6) at 30 dB relative to SL bilaterally (i.e., 30 dB relative to better ear), with ambient narrow-band masking level (500 Hz) at 30 dB relative to SL. Masking should be calibrated with filter in the out position.
Criterion: response control criterion (5/0).

Phase 13.
Increase masking level by 10 dB.
Criterion: response control criterion (5/0).

Phase 14. Masking and S^D Generalization
Generalize to other frequencies (order 1 KHz, 2 KHz, 4 KHz, and 250 Hz) with appropriate narrow-band masking at 20 dB below S^D and S^D at 30 dB relative to SL for each frequency.
Criterion: two consecutive responses (2/0) at each frequency before proceeding to next frequency. If the subject misses two consecutive responses, return to the previously successful frequency. If he still is unsuccessful, use a greater difference between masking and S^D.

Phase 15.

It now is assumed that the subject has completed pretraining masking procedures and is ready for masked auditory thresholds. Assess thresholds by standard procedures and by the descending threshold technique.

LITERATURE CITED

Carhart, R. and J. F. Jerger. 1959. Preferred method for clinical determination of pure-tone thresholds. J. Speech Hear. Dis. 24: 330–345.
Studebaker, G. A. 1964. Clinical masking of air- and bone-conduction stimuli. J. Speech Hear. Dis. 29: 23–35.

B Reinforcement Delivery Apparatus and Response Mechanism

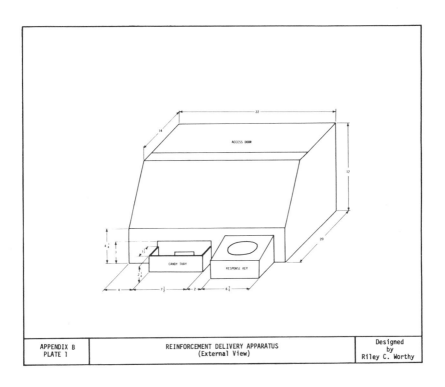

APPENDIX B PLATE 1	REINFORCEMENT DELIVERY APPARATUS (External View)	Designed by Riley C. Worthy

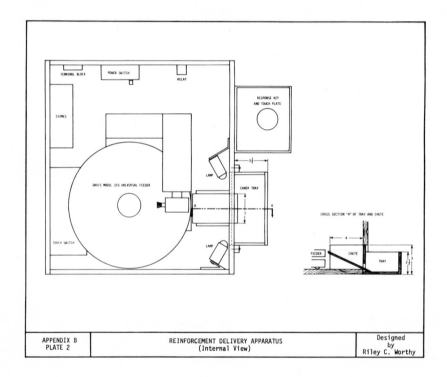

| APPENDIX B PLATE 2 | REINFORCEMENT DELIVERY APPARATUS (Internal View) | Designed by Riley C. Worthy |

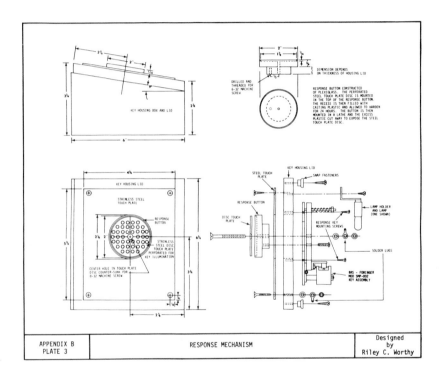

RESPONSE MECHANISM

Designed
by
Riley C. Worthy

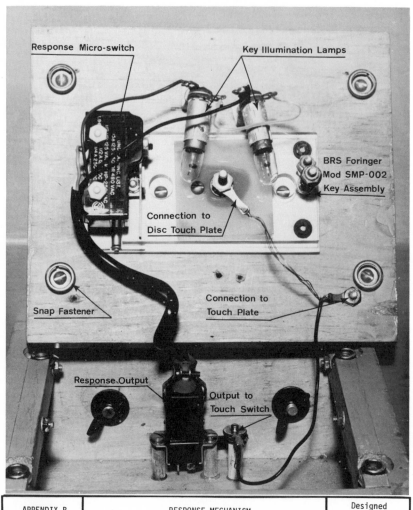

| APPENDIX B
PLATE 4 | RESPONSE MECHANISM
(Bottom View) | Designed
by
Riley C. Worthy |

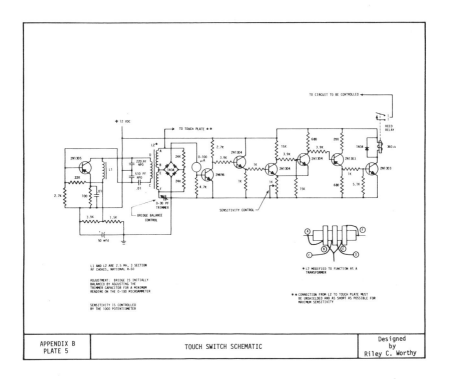

| APPENDIX B
PLATE 5 | TOUCH SWITCH SCHEMATIC | Designed
by
Riley C. Worthy |

C Puretone and SISI Programming Schematics

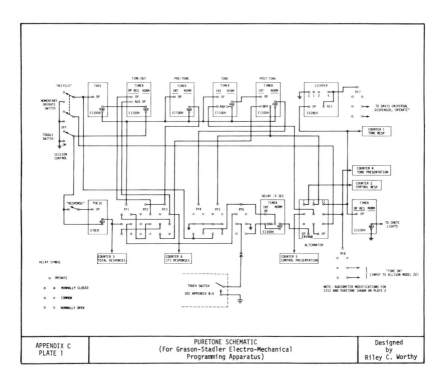

APPENDIX C PLATE 1	PURETONE SCHEMATIC (For Grason-Stadler Electro-Mechanical Programming Apparatus)	Designed by Riley C. Worthy

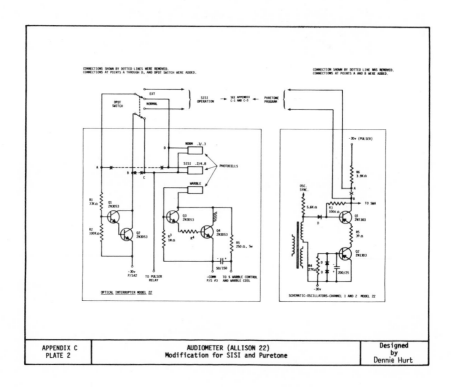

| APPENDIX C
PLATE 2 | AUDIOMETER (ALLISON 22)
Modification for SISI and Puretone | Designed
by
Dennie Hurt |

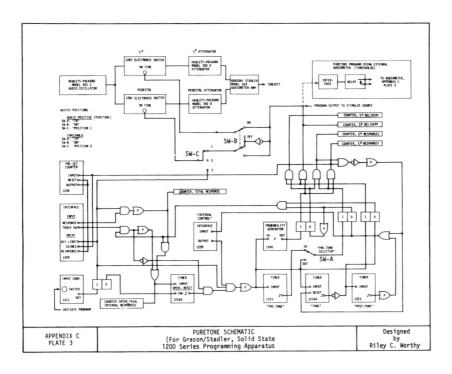

APPENDIX C
PLATE 3

PURETONE SCHEMATIC
(For Grason/Stadler, Solid State
1200 Series Programming Apparatus

Designed
by
Riley C. Worthy

D Tone Decay Programming Schematic

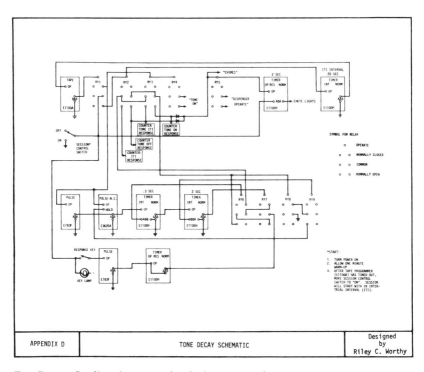

| APPENDIX D | TONE DECAY SCHEMATIC | Designed by Riley C. Worthy |

For Grason-Stadler electromechanical programming apparatus

E Short-Duration Programming Schematic

The short-duration augmentation and short-duration interruption studies were controlled by the puretone program schematic shown in Appendix C, Plate 3, with control settings as follows for short-duration interruption:

Switch A, "out"
Switch B, "on"
Switch C, Position 3

and short-duration augmentation:

Switches A and C same as above
Switch B in "off" position

F Frequency DL Programming Schematic

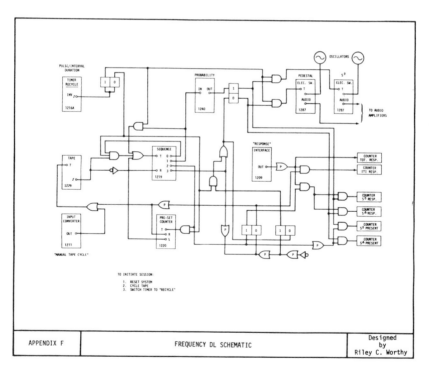

APPENDIX F	FREQUENCY DL SCHEMATIC	Designed by Riley C. Worthy

For Grason-Stadler 1200 series solid state programming apparatus

G Intensity-Increment Programming Schematic

The intensity study program was controlled by the puretone program schematic in Appendix C, Plate 3, with Switch A at the "in" position, Switch B "on," and Switch C in Position 3. The S^D attenuator is replaced with a nonstandard one constructed to produce 0.2-dB increments.

Author Index

Subject Index

Acoustic signals (parameters of). *See* Duration; Frequency; Intensity
Adaptation, 68–70
Air Conduction, 6. *See also* Thresholds
Amplitude Modulation, 111
Animal Research, 3
Anticipation factor, 49
Apparatus. *See* Instrumentation
Auditory training. *See* Earphone training
Augmentation Detection. *See* Detection

Behavioral audiometry, 14
Bone Conduction, 6. *See also* Thresholds
Bridging stimuli. *See* Stimuli
Button. *See* Switch

Capacitance Switch. *See* Switch
Carry-over, 32–33
Conditioned orientation reflex audiometry, 17
Conditioned reinforcers. *See* Reinforcers
Conditioning instrumental/Operant, 13, 14
Controls, 23, 83, 85, 87, 105, 136
  Control events, 105
  Control periods, 23, 83, 85, 87, 105, 136

Cortical-evoked response, 1
Cortical Lesions, 7
Criterion, 23, 24, 30–32, 39–44, 57, 71–72, 104, 113, 115
  Stimulus-response control criterion, 23, 24, 39–44, 71–72

Detection, 7, 82–96, 111–118
  Augmentation, 82–92
  Intensity, 111–118
  Interruption, 92–96
  Stimulus change, 7
Difference limen, 81, 97–109, 111–118, 155, 157
  Frequency, 97–109, **155**
  Intensity, 81, 111–118, 157
Discrete response, 17, 19
Discriminative stimulus. *See* Stimuli
Dispensers. *See* Instrumentation
Drugs, 5
Duration, 57, 81, 86, 93, 113, 136–137, 153
  Detection, 86
  Equivalent, 86, 113
  Stimulus, 57, 86, 137

Earphone training, 20–21, 134
Extinction, 48

Fading, 20, 138
Formants, 109, 111, 126